CANCER HATES TEA

A Unique Preventive and Transformative
Lifestyle Change to Help *Crush Cancer*

Maria Uspenski

Founder of The Tea Spot

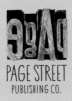

PAGE STREET
PUBLISHING CO.

PAGE STREET
PUBLISHING CO.

Copyright © 2016 Maria Uspenski

First published in 2016 by

Page Street Publishing Co.

27 Congress Street, Suite 1511

Salem, MA 01970

www.pagestreetpublishing.com

Distributed by Macmillan, sales in Canada by The Canadian Manda Group.

27 26 25 24 23   9 10 11 12 13

ISBN-13: 978-1-62414-312-0

ISBN-10: 1-62414-312-1

Library of Congress Control Number: 2016940211

Cover and book design by Page Street Publishing Co.

Photography by Ted Axelrod

Cover Photography and Illustrations by Hope Larsen

Printed and bound in the United States

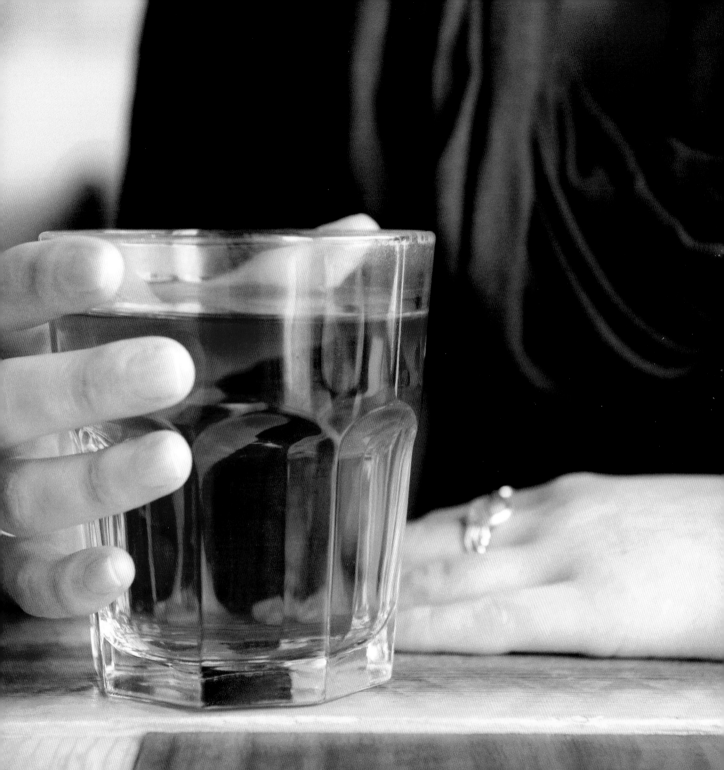

Dedicated to Pirate, the most extraordinary cancer fighter.

CONTENTS

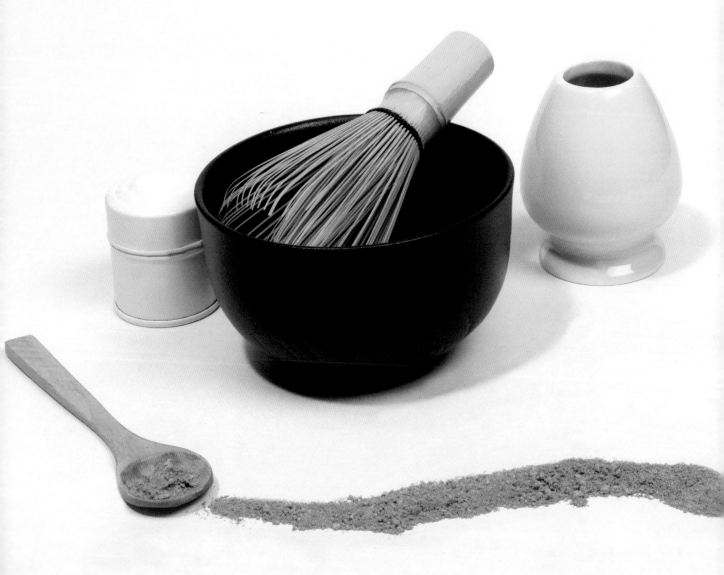

FOREWORD by Dr. Mary L. Hardy

The "big four" cancers in the United States are breast, prostate, colon/rectal and lung cancer. These four sites alone will account for almost 1.7 million new cases of cancer this year. Add to that the 15.5 million cancer survivors already worrying about recurrence and you have a lot of people looking for ways to make themselves more cancer unfriendly.

Some risk factors we can't modify but happily **everyone** can make changes that significantly reduce their chances of hearing those three scary words—"You have cancer." What you eat and drink, how much you move and how you manage stress are under **your** control and can account for up to 85% of your risk. Smart choices in these areas create the key components of a comprehensive wellness program.

However, it can be overwhelming to put together a practical program out of all the confusing information available in the media. Luckily, you are holding in your hand a very useful tool to give cancer a kick in the pants. Maria Uspenski, herself a cancer survivor, has taken her personal experience and extensive knowledge and crafted a clear plan for you to follow.

She starts by filling in a lot of technical background about cancer, how it starts and how it grows and spreads so that you can understand the context for the healthy habits she promotes in this book. Scientific information is interspersed with charming historical facts and practical tips that make prevention feel achievable. The advice in this book is grounded in research but is made more compelling by her feisty attitude and personal passion for wellness.

The major focus of this book is tea and that is a smart move. Since the first tea leaves drifted into the cup of a long ago Chinese emperor, the heavenly elixir has been associated with health. The scientific literature shows over 1,300 human clinical trials on health effects of tea including results in cancer risk reduction, increasing heart health, metabolic modification and improving liver health. The chemical components of tea: polyphenols, amino acid and caffeine, have dozens of anti-cancer mechanisms. She also shows how tea can impact other healthy habits such as weight control, heart health and meditation.

Although tea is the second most popular beverage in the world after water, the American public is still not very familiar with the rich variety of teas available from tea plantations across the globe. Maria's depth of knowledge of the various types of teas and the proper methods of preparation is deep. You will learn about the most powerful tea for cancer prevention, green tea and the most antioxidant-rich version of green tea, matcha. But green tea will be just the beginning. She describes the full range of tea, from white through oolong to black and pu-erh. Shorter sections on key herbal teas are included as well.

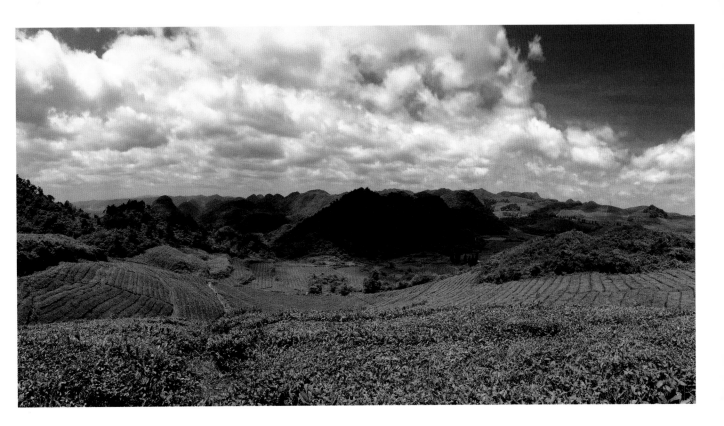

Through information about healthy diet, exercise and stress management as well as the detailed information about optimal preparation of tea, she helps you set specific goals and outlines practical strategies to meet these goals. Since the best cup of tea is the one you are willing to drink, she provides guidance to a wide variety of choices so that you can find the tea variety and preparation method that best suits you and your health goals. This transforms tea drinking from a dutiful chore into a healthy pleasure.

So let's raise a cup to toast your commitment to improving your health. Enjoy this excellent guide along your journey.

To our good health and to the joys of full bodied living,

Mary L. Hardy, MD
Former Medical Director of Simms/Mann UCLA Center for Integrative Oncology
Founder, Wellness Works

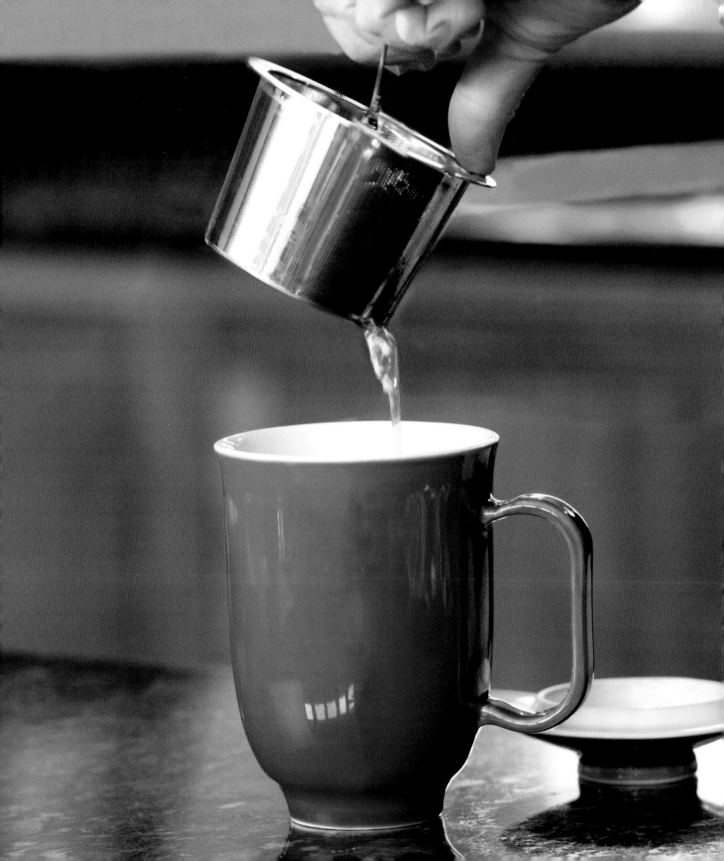

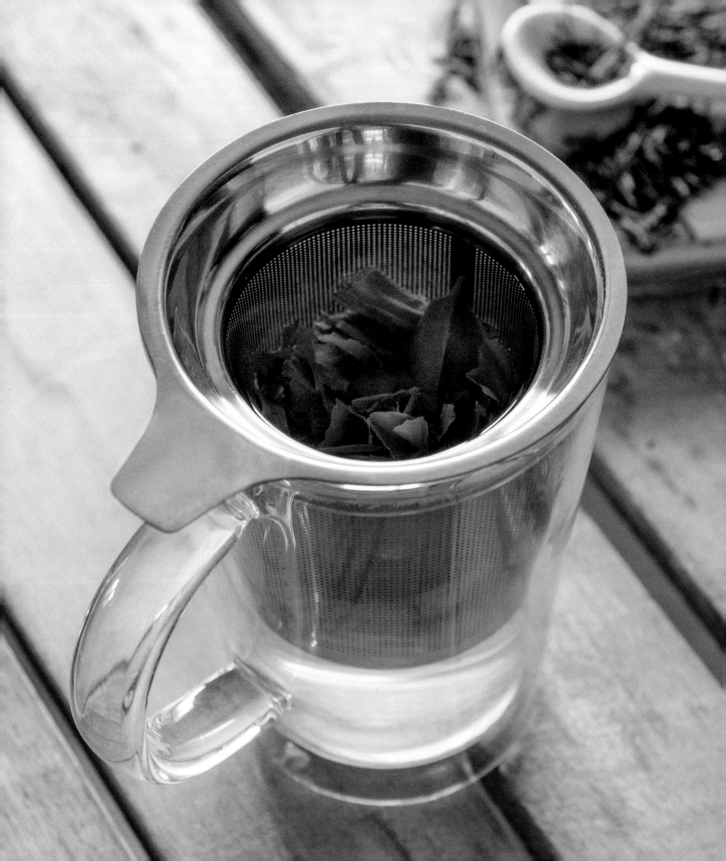

INTRODUCTION

Cancer monumentally sucks. Cancer attacks people you love. Cancer destroys beautiful lives. Cancer takes away our loved ones. Cancer likes to act as though it's more invincible than we are.

When I was first told about my cancer diagnosis, I thought it had to be a mistake. I felt like I was all of a sudden inhabiting someone else's body, or dreaming. I thought to myself that clearly, I just needed to get myself out of the doctor's office in order for everything to be fine again. I asked to see the data and have it explained, and then proceeded to ask for more tests and to get other opinions. Surely, I thought, this couldn't be my reality—I was athletic, a non-smoker and in my prime, or so I thought. All I could think of were my young daughters and that they needed me. The first thing I wanted to do was race home and enjoy our daily after-school snack and chat. I knew this act of normalcy would ground me and would get me calm enough to start working through how to deal with this fast treadmill of disease management I now found myself on. I was young and naïve enough to not even consider a sad outcome.

As it turned out, with amazing medical and healing care, much love and just plain pushing through on my part, I made the transition from cancer patient to having "no evidence of disease." I've never understood why I was one of the lucky ones in my experience with cancer, but once I had arrived at that monumental threshold, I wasn't ready to just forget and party on. That piece-of-crap disease had almost managed to wrench me away from my young children for good. With my new remission status, I turned my focus 100 percent onto preventing the recurrence of this rotten threat, which I felt was still haunting me and constantly breathing down my neck. It took me years to get to the point where I finally felt safe enough to ignore the whispers of doubt in my head and get to a point where I was not constantly listening and sensing signs of recurrence. During this recovery I read every study I could get my hands on about maintaining cancer wellness. Because I'm an analytical person by background, I wanted to know every process of how cancer grows, to understand what prompted those biochemical mechanisms to begin with and find out what could possibly thwart them.

In my research, I found the most compelling evidence advocated for a five-cup-a-day (1.2 L) tea habit. In this book, I will show you how you can make this powerful routine a part of your every day without turning your life upside down or your wallet inside out. It's an encapsulation of all I've learned about the health benefits of tea as an anti-cancer food on my adventure along the road to wellness, post-disease. Part One of the book is a basic primer on both cancer and tea chemistry. In becoming well-informed on the powers of the tea leaf, it helps to appreciate the seriousness of the cancer beast on a cellular level, as well as how our immune systems work. Part Two conveys practical information on making your own tea, how much and when to drink it, and how to make this change to your routine effortless and straightforward. Part Three presents additional anti-cancer actions and the teas that can help on the journey toward achieving your best possible state of immunity. In Part Four of the book, you'll find all the how-to's to help in choosing your first teas and a plan you can follow for guidance to get into the tea-fit groove, more advanced information on teas (for when you're hooked!) and some recipes that will help you pull tea into your diet.

Tea, and in particular green tea, came up time and time again in most everything I came across related to cancer health. How I would have loved to have been a student of Thomas Edison a century ago, when he predicted, "The doctor of the future will give no medicine, but will interest his patient in the care of the human frame—in diet and in the cause and prevention of disease." The consensus common to many of the research studies I found on tea and cancer was that drinking five servings of tea daily could have a significant effect on reducing the incidence and growth of cancerous tumors. So drink tea I did—with intensity. I sourced full leaf green teas since these were touted to be the anti-cancer specialists in virtually all the studies I'd come across. I drank like my life depended on it.

Tea is the most studied anti-cancer plant. Over the past 10 years, more than 5,000 medical studies have been published on the health benefits of tea, with over 1,000 of those focusing specifically on tea and cancer. The National Institutes of Health's stance on green tea is that research indicates it to be possibly effective against many afflictions, including several types of cancer, clogged arteries, osteoporosis and Parkinson's disease. It also states that it's likely safe for adults to drink five cups a day. I found it paradoxical that my most potent defense against cancer was apparently within my own control and was already growing right in nature's backyard. "Let food be thy medicine and medicine be thy food," advocated Hippocrates 2,000 years ago. I learned I could create the ideal diet for restoring and maintaining wellness, simply by eliminating refined and processed foods from my diet.

If cancer doesn't like the playing field in your body, it will retreat.

Since that time over 10 years ago, I've continued to pursue answers by making wellness my life's work and have extended my efforts beyond my own health to that of my daughters, other young women and basically anyone I can reach. I studied for a certification in fitness nutrition and started a tea company where our mission is to foster wellness through tea. We handcraft our own whole leaf tea blends and source more than 100 teas and herbals from around the globe. I use my engineering background in my work to design what I call 'Steepware'—cups, filters, teapots and bottles that make the preparation and serving of loose leaf tea easy.

My goal is to relate in an easily digestible format what I've learned and experienced about how tea works when it helps your body's defenses. I'm not a medical professional and no statement in this book should be interpreted as direction or prescription. In my simplistic explanations, I in no way mean to make light of the serious research that forms the basis for the understanding of the biological mechanisms of how the body responds to disease. References and sources for specific tea health statements throughout the book are included in the References (page 202), so you can pursue further reading on the subject.

It's not easy, dealing with that rotten monster cancer. It not only messes with your body, it does some serious damage to your mind—at least it did with mine. I know I was a pretty good mess. Fortunately, I had a few close, smart, kick-ass friends who would not allow me to give up. With their guidance and insistence, I was able to grasp on to little tidbits of the many turning points which I firmly believe helped me through. To this day I cannot articulate without tears that out of the five women in my first support group I am the only one left standing. That truth forces me to fully realize that today, tomorrow, next month and next year are never ensured. My cancer journey brought me to a vital realization that my every day is the most important day. For the past ten-plus years on this journey, drinking five cups of tea has been a constant and non-negotiable priority of my every day.

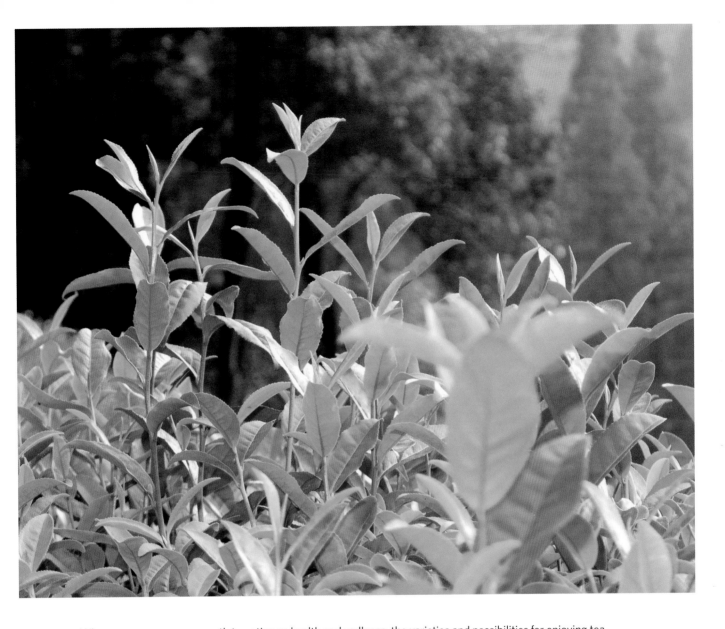

Wherever you are on your path to optimum health and wellness, the varieties and possibilities for enjoying tea are endless. The great news is that the effects of drinking tea daily can start making a measurable difference in your body in as little as six weeks. Don't deprive yourself—why not work to level the playing field more to your advantage? A batter can't wait for the ball to cross home plate before deciding whether it's something to swing at. Nor should you. Don't wait for cancer to strike you with a speedy curveball before you begin.

Steep.

-PART ONE-

WHY CANCER
HATES
TEA

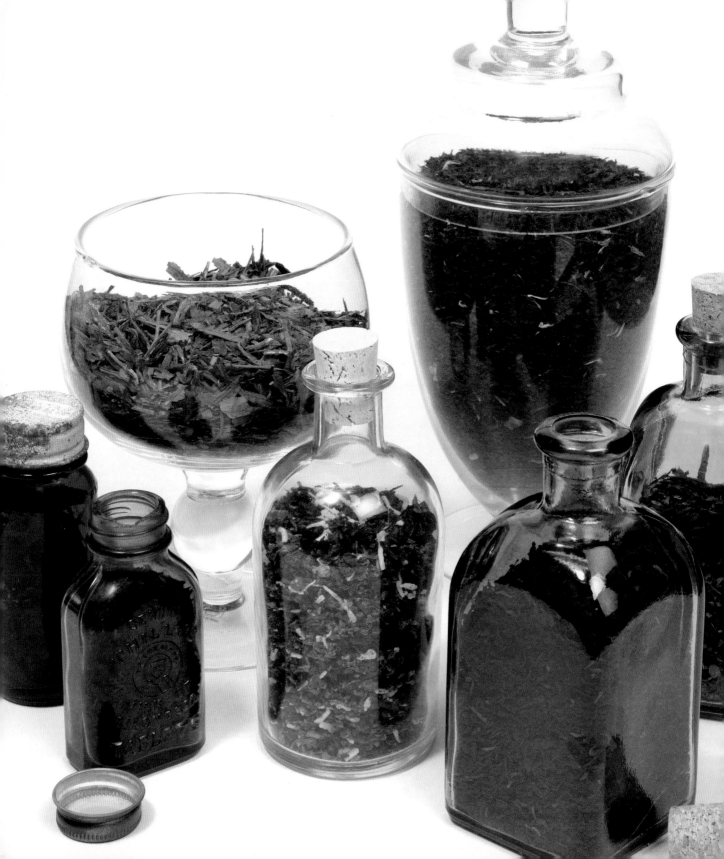

Chapter 1

CANCER 101—HOW IT WORKS

KNOWLEDGE IS POWER

What is Cancer Anyway?

*Let's get something straight right off the bat: **Cancer isn't something you catch.** It's not like the flu that gets passed around the family, or something you can prevent by washing your hands. Cancer is something that gets triggered within your own body. Its initiation begins with a single screw-up in a cell's genetic code—which can go awry for any number of reasons, including stress, poor diet, smoking, sun exposure, toxins in the environment, even just plain life and aging. Having one or more risk factors doesn't mean that cancer is on its way—it can't survive on its own. It actually needs to be promoted, with your help, in order to succeed against you. Cancer works like an opportunistic scavenging empire builder, feeding right off your own body.*

*Good news: Your immune system is programmed to not let that happen and more often than not it's a top-notch cancer killing SWAT team. **Your body stares into the face of death and saves your life daily.** Of the trillions of cells alive inside you now, many thousands of them are downright nasty dudes, with the ability to seriously mess some things up in the marvelous landscape that is your physiology. Your immune system is busy keeping tabs on millions of cells 24/7. It knows exactly when to yell "Die now!" selectively putting an end to those potentially damaging cells before they get a chance to do any harm. This enormously powerful scenario plays out thousands of times each and every day. You are one beautiful piece of machinery.*

Bad news: Sometimes, those detrimental cells manage to get past your protective squad. This happens when your immune system gets tricked by some cancerous monsters or it's just overwhelmed on too many fronts to put up a good fight. Cancer begins slowly and surreptitiously, with just one or a small group of mutated cells, but not for long. The pace at which cancer cells divide and multiply cascades like an avalanche, progressing until they form together in a wicked organized group— a malignant tumor. Its malicious goal is to spread over as many parts of your human organism as it possibly can. Then your body's left dealing with this invasive monster—much like a pine tree contending with beetle kill. And that is absolutely no joke.

***Understanding cancer is difficult.** Wrapping your head around how something as simple as tea could have any legitimate effect on cancer is also difficult. This chapter breaks it down step-by-step, and molecule-by-molecule, so as to allow you to understand what cellular mechanisms are happening when that tricky bastard cancer meets up with tea.*

Let's steep on.

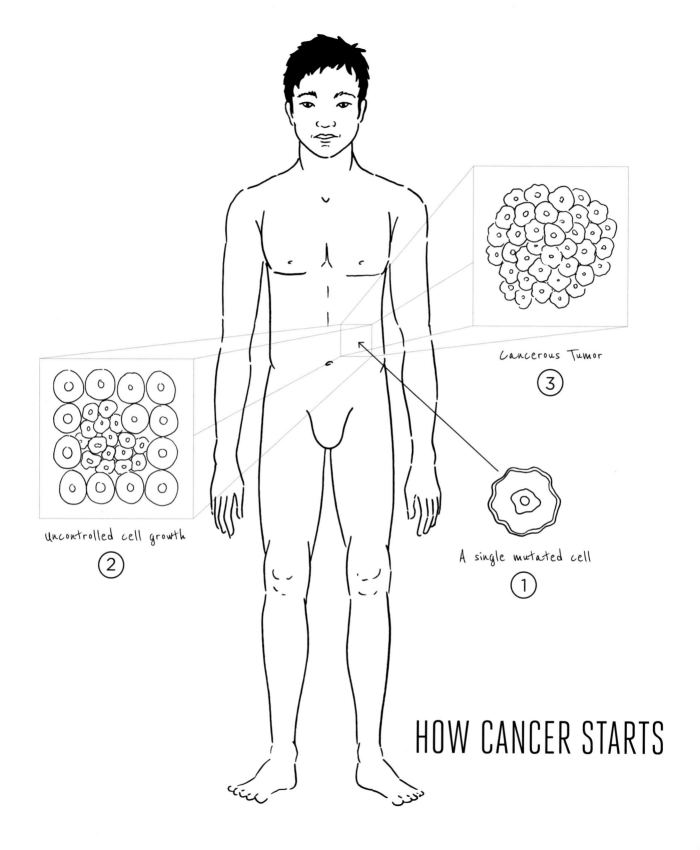

Cancerous Tumor

③

Uncontrolled cell growth

②

A single mutated cell

①

HOW CANCER STARTS

THE CRAZINESS THAT IS CANCER

Cancer is a term used for more than 100 different diseases that can start just about anywhere in your body. Each one of those diseases is distinct and works to destroy in unique ways, but they all have these three characteristics in common:

ABNORMAL CELLS THAT MULTIPLY WITHOUT CONTROL

Every day, millions of cells divide, grow and develop to produce more cells in your body. In babies and children, cells divide rapidly to support the growth of the organism. By the time we're adults this cell division slows down. Cancer cell growth is different from normal cell growth in that cancer cells replicate faster, without any respect for the meticulous order your body is wired for. What's key here is that we're talking about rapid growth of abnormal cells. They multiply faster than heck, they resist destruction in the natural course of cell death and they can overwhelm your immune system and normal healthy cells.

GROWTH AND PROLIFERATION THAT DESTROYS SURROUNDING TISSUES

Because cancer cells are multiplying more rapidly, they're consuming more of your cells' energy reserves. If a microscopic cancer gets its start without being shut down, it will keep growing and begin to form a tumor. This requires oxygen for energy, which the cancer coerces your body into supplying by getting it to build blood vessels to deliver oxygen to the tumor-building site. Once those blood vessels are created, the cancer can invade surrounding tissues.

THE ABILITY TO SPREAD TO DISTANT ORGANS IN THE BODY

This unique ability is what makes cancer so ridiculously scary. When a tumor sits nicely contained in isolation somewhere in your body, it can simply be removed. Cancer is a conniving disease, though, and by invading tissues and spreading throughout your body, it is much more of a challenge to hunt down and arrest. This is cancer's end game, and you've undoubtedly heard of it—metastasis.

Cancer is pure chaos. How does anything as wildly out of control as this disease ever get past your highly organized and systemized immune system?

There's no single cause of cancer, although there are a number of underlying risk factors, such as getting too many ultraviolet rays from the sun or exposure to cigarette smoke and other toxins.

The scary thing is that people with several risk factors might never develop the disease, whereas others who do develop cancer didn't have any of the known risk factors. To make matters more complicated, different cancers have different risk factors, and different cancers behave differently. Some people have super slow-growing cancers which they manage like a chronic disease, while others have cancers which can turn their life upside down within weeks. While some risk factors can actually provoke the onset of cancer, others (such as old age) might just be more common in people who get cancer.

Even with all of that unexplained craziness, there are a number of mitigating steps that can be taken to lessen your risk of cancer. Health organizations worldwide estimate that at least one-third of all cancer cases could be prevented. One well-referenced study from The University of Texas M.D. Anderson Cancer Center points out that since only 5–10 percent of all cancer cases can be attributed to genetic predisposition that the remaining 90–95 percent have their roots in lifestyle and environment. That's downright mind-blowing, isn't it? The onset of the cancer monster, which is responsible for one in every four deaths in the U.S., can be prevented. Why isn't everyone standing in line for that?

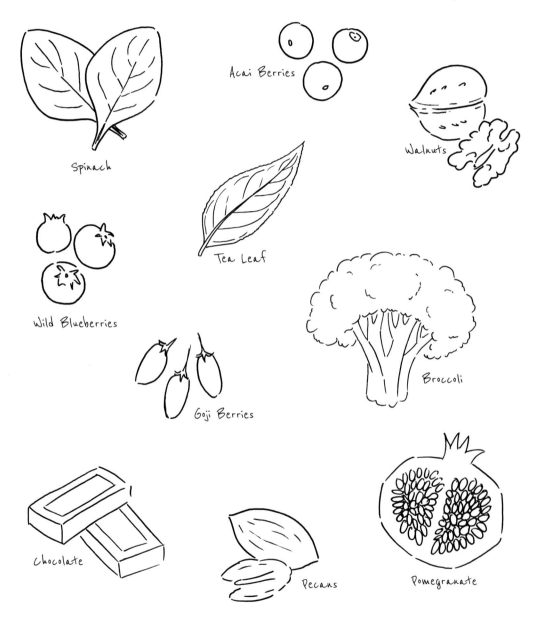

Spinach

Acai Berries

Walnuts

Tea Leaf

Wild Blueberries

Broccoli

Goji Berries

Chocolate

Pecans

Pomegranate

FOODS HIGH IN POLYPHENOL ANTIOXIDANTS

HOW CANCER BEGINS

Cancer is lurking everywhere. All animals and even plants can get cancer. People of any age can get cancer and it can develop anywhere in your body. The average human body is made up of tens of trillions of cells. Those trillions of living, dying, growing and dividing cells require consummate order and organization. Their management has to happen in a very specific and controlled manner. When your body's cells become defective, they die and you regenerate healthy cells. In fact, you shed the equivalent of your total body weight in dead cells each year. When you're healthy, the birth and death of each cell is carefully controlled so that every part of you always has just the right number of cells. This process is guided by your genetic blueprint commander-in-chief deoxyribonucleic acid (DNA). It's present in each and every one of your cells and contains your entire genetic makeup. DNA is essential for telling the cells in your body how to behave.

Everyone inevitably sustains physiological strain to their cells each and every day, either as a result of the chemical processes going on to keep you alive and kicking, or because you're fighting inflammation or noxious invaders such as tobacco smoke and ultra-violet (UV) rays. This brings on a damaging cellular condition known as oxidative stress, which produces chemically unstable molecules, called free radicals, in your body. Under optimal operating conditions, your immune system can deal with just bashing them out. But there are instances when your immune system might not be able to keep up with counteracting the effects of oxidative stress and all the free radicals being generated in your body, and this creates an imbalance favoring the onslaught of those highly reactive molecules, which can have harmful effects on your cells' DNA. Your body's biochemical mechanism for counteracting free radicals is to neutralize them with antioxidants. At the deepest cellular level, antioxidants stop free radicals dead in their tracks by stabilizing them chemically, before those reactive agents can chemically attack your cells' DNA. Left unmanaged in their highly reactive state, free radicals can cause your DNA to spontaneously change its genetic message. This makes the cell no longer part of you, but a strange and screwed up mutation of you, evil doppelgänger style.

Ordinarily, the cells under attack repair their own DNA. It's estimated that an individual cell can fix up to a million changes to its DNA every day. When it doesn't get repaired, your immune system lets these mutations know they're not welcome, inviting them to gracefully die off. If one of the damaged cells doesn't die off, that mutation can continue to replicate with messed up DNA, and that's where real trouble can set in. The genesis of cancer is due to that key genetic change to the DNA in your cells. Eventually, the strangely mutated cells will spawn a whole new hoard of cells, all with mutated DNA, and they don't behave according to your body's original master plan. Their mutated progeny are very high energy and may begin to act immortal in your body, since they're not playing by your rulebook. An accumulation of mutated cells will progressively go on transforming the cells outside your normal DNA code. Most of the time, damaged cells will eventually stop reproducing on their own, or form harmless, benign tumors. But in some cases they can keep growing ravenously out of control, becoming malignant. And that spells C-A-N-C-E-R.

NATURE'S CANCER NEUTRALIZERS

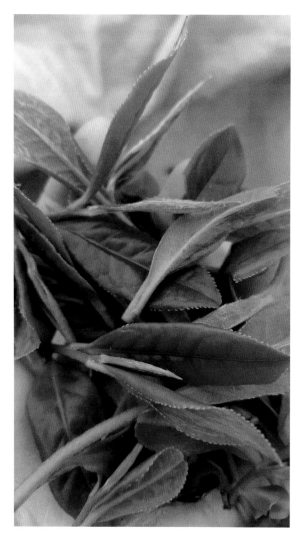

When cancer's battling on unfriendly terrain, it can be forced to pump the brakes or retreat altogether. Your immune system fights cancer on multiple fronts and at every phase of its progression, beginning even before its inception, when free radicals are just beginning to cause chemical instability in your cells. Over the past several decades, we've seen a lot of attention on free radical chemistry, because those rascals can trigger a lot of human diseases. Your body needs to keep the balance between antioxidants and free radicals in your favor in order to maintain proper physiological function. As it turns out, cancer has its weaknesses—antioxidants are its very own Achilles' heel. So where do these antioxidants come from?

Plants aren't equipped with an immune system like we are, but they're good at standing their ground against extreme environmental factors, bacterial organisms and invading critters. A plant has its own set of biochemical defenses that it depends on for its daily survival. Those are the same chemical defenders that come to our aid when we ingest plant material. As soon as a plant comes under attack, its DNA activates this army of defenders to wage chemical warfare. It can help protect the plant from threats as wide-ranging as UV radiation, disease, invading microorganisms and competing plants. Threatening pests find these chemical combatants bitter and distasteful. This is interesting because these distasteful attributes are the same compounds that provide the astringent tastes we've come to love in tea. These powerful warrior compounds are polyphenol antioxidants and they soldier through our cells, sacrificing themselves by neutralizing hazardous molecules gone awry. Polyphenol antioxidants are like the star players who help the immune system team play at its peak in this game.

Enter your own personal army: the tea leaf, a most powerful natural source of antioxidants.

ANTIOXIDANTS AT WORK

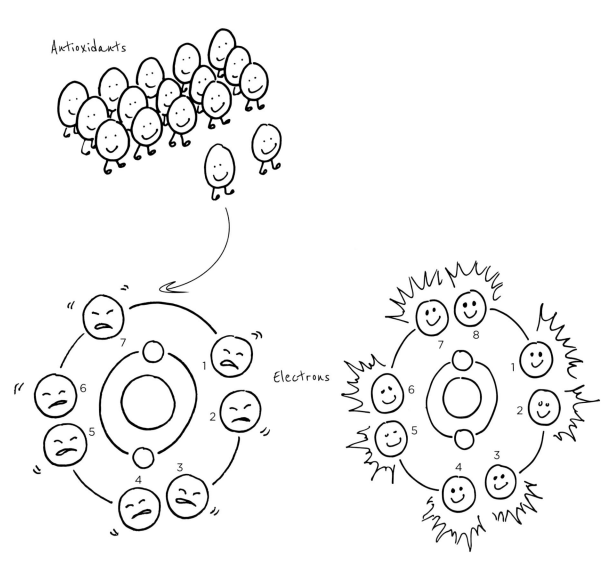

Antioxidants

Electrons

Raging Free Radical: Only seven electrons in the outer ring, this configuration is unstable, UH OH!

Neutralized Free Radical: Electron donated by an antioxidant gives outer ring eight electrons, this configuration is stable, YEAH!

WHY TEA?

The term "survivor" doesn't sit well with me. As strong as I feel today, I know those cancer cells currently dormant inside me just might break into a wild rave without giving me notice, calling my body back into a seriously bad romance which I have absolutely no desire to revisit. I was lucky enough to make it through a battle, but there is no guarantee that the war is over; not for me, not for anyone.

But why tea? Why not go crazy on other antioxidant-rich choices such as blueberries, pomegranates, or better yet, dark chocolate and red wine? Tea ranks higher than most fruits and vegetables in antioxidant potential and Vitamins C and K content. In all the studies I've read, there's a strong relationship between antioxidants and anti-inflammation, immune system function and anti-cancer activities in the human body. I've come to agree with the science that claims that cancer is a largely preventable disease and that the function of the immune system and cancer are in inextricably linked. Various medical studies from many different countries around the world have reported on tea as an anti-inflammation agent, as well as a selective immune-system booster in pursuing selective anti-cancer mechanisms. Note: In this book I don't refer to studies done on mice, as legitimate as they may be. I'm just not educated enough to make the jump from how something works in a mouse to how it would work in my own body.

I've always loved tea, but over the past decade, I've learned to appreciate great teas and their amazing health benefits more than I would have ever thought possible. One of the things I liked about tea is that it's a plant-based substance that exhibits some of those same selective biochemical actions as promising newer targeted cancer therapies and therefore looked like a non-toxic anti-cancer agent. If something as simple and natural as tea could help make any progress in regressing any cancerous activity and reducing the risk of recurrence, even indirectly, I was all in. It seemed to me like a win-win. So here we are. I hate cancer. I'm not leaving it all up to tea, but as an integral and consistent part of my diet and commitment to regular exercise, I view it as an added insurance policy in helping mobilize my body's immune system against cancer. It's become a simple and affordable daily luxury, and the fact that I love the taste, the ceremony and how it makes me feel, are just added benefits.

TEA, DEFINED

Not everything we dunk in water and drink as tea is actually tea, biologically speaking. The dictionary gives us a slew of definitions for *tea*, and these give us insight as to how loosely the term is used and why it can sometimes be confusing:

1. A hot drink made by infusing the dried, crushed leaves of the tea plant in boiling water.
2. The dried leaves used to make tea.
3. A drink made from the infused leaves, fruits or flowers of plants other than tea. Herbal tea or fruit tea.
4. Any hot drink, for example, coffee or cocoa.
5. The evergreen shrub or small tree that produces tea leaves, native to southern and eastern Asia and grown as a major cash crop.
6. A light afternoon meal consisting typically of tea to drink, sandwiches and cakes.
7. A cooked evening meal.
8. Breakfast, typically consisting of a hot drink and bread.

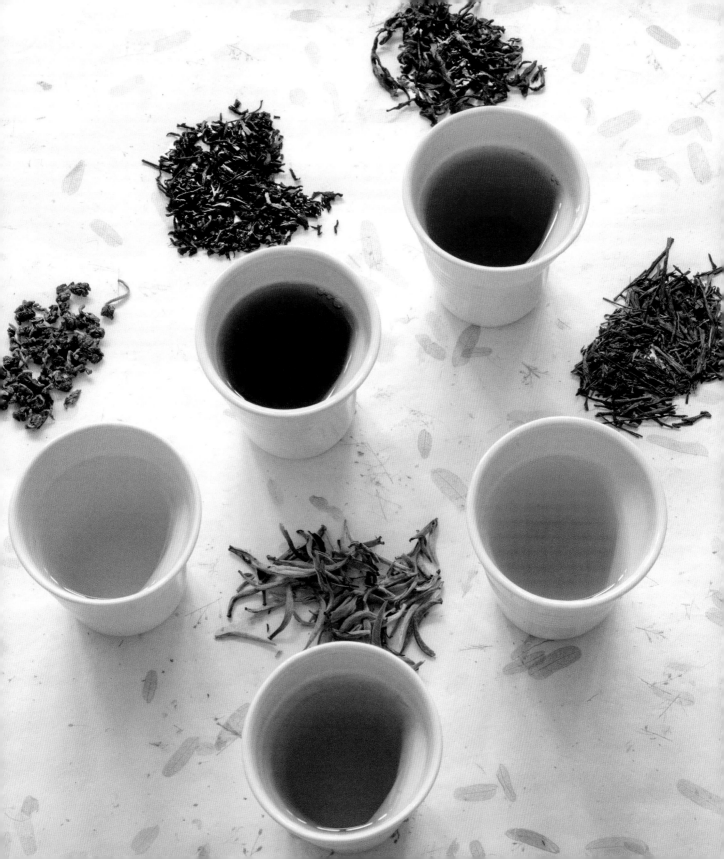

We're going to stick with the first two definitions only and discuss tea as the finished leaf product of the tea plant, *Camellia sinensis* or its water extract.

Tea is so simple; really, it's just leaf and water. It quenches our thirst and helps keep us hydrated. But once a tea drinker learns to appreciate the many nuances of flavor the tea leaf can embody, he or she is on their way to an amazing sensory voyage. Most cultures around the world have made tea part of their daily ritual, not because of its healing properties, but as a celebration of its culinary, aesthetic and mood-lifting qualities. Simply put, tea is one of life's pleasures. It makes people feel better and provides a quick, relaxing escape from life's hectic pace. This 5,000-year-old infusion is the most consumed beverage on the planet after water.

The history of medicinal herbs is rich and diverse and even older than that of tea. It includes many things we call tea, such as peppermint, chamomile and hibiscus, but strictly speaking, they're not really tea. They're herbals, fruits or florals. What we're focused on here are the leaves that come from the *Camellia sinensis* plant. These leaves possess the unique tea health benefits we're chasing. Teas made from this plant are classified under four main tea types: white/green, oolong, black and pu-erh. The customary way to make a tea beverage is by infusing its dried leaves into hot water, and this remains the most popular way of consuming tea today.

HOW *CAMELLIA* BECOMES TEA

Camellia sinensis (the meaning in Latin is "Chinese Camellia") is native to Southeast Asia, and now cultivated in more than 30 countries. This single species of plant yields more than 9 billion pounds (4,000 kilotonnes) of finished tea each year. Thanks to different varietals of the plant, production methods, growing and harvest season, and soil and weather conditions, one tea species produces a wildly broad range of flavors and appearances. How is it possible that a delicate and calming green tea comes from the same botanical as a nectarous and mysterious black tea? It all really comes down to the chemical process of oxidation.

Tea leaves, like all plant matter, are made up of mostly water. As soon as they're picked off the tea plant, they start to wilt. With time and exposure to air they dehydrate and start to turn brown, or oxidize, just like any other fresh leaves would, or like a cut apple turns brown. This happens as a result of a series of enzyme-driven chemical processes in the leaves. Oxidation (no relation to oxidative stress in your cells) can be enhanced by manually manipulating, rolling and crushing the tea leaves. When leaves get to the desired level of oxidation for the type of tea that's being produced, the process is stopped by using heat to dry the tea out completely, killing the oxidative enzymes in the leaves and halting any further oxidative action. From that point on, the tea leaves are chemically stable and they don't change or evolve any further. What you have then is your final tea product. A longer oxidation period in the tea manufacturing process makes the leaves darker and gives them more of the traditional characteristic black tea flavor and aroma. The type of tea that *Camellia sinensis* turns into is entirely a function of how much oxidation it undergoes during processing.

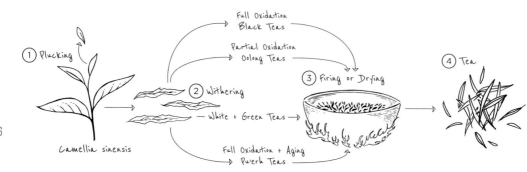

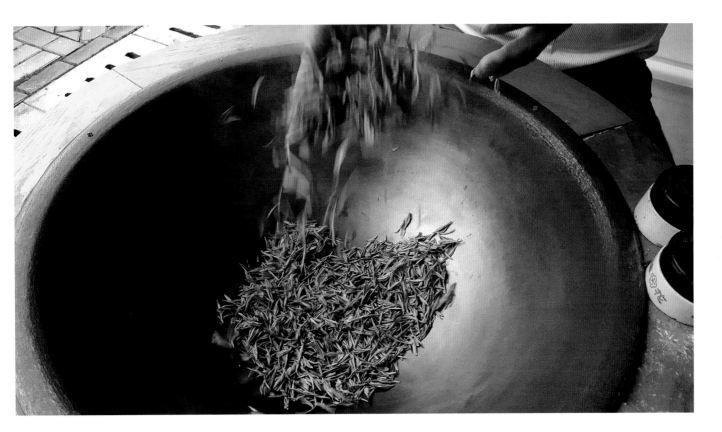

For the four basic types of tea products manufactured, oxidation levels range from "not at all" (white/green) to "max-plus" (pu-erh).

White/Green — White teas are the closest thing to a fresh tea leaf, and they look that way—leafy and downy. Green tea is produced by pan-firing or steaming tea leaves which have not been oxidized, which is why the tea retains a fresher green color. They have a more subtle, astringent taste than darker teas, but they pack a mean antioxidant punch.

Oolong — Oolong teas span the widest oxidation range of all the tea types, ranging in levels from very little to almost as much as a black tea. Oolongs are complex, which makes them fun. They can look and taste very close to a green tea, or be as dark as a black tea, but with unexpected notes of a lighter tea. Grown primarily in China and Taiwan, they are partially oxidized before being rolled and then pan fired to finish treatment.

Black — Black tea is made from crushed tea leaves which have been through an enzyme-driven oxidation period. They've been given the time and air to wither and fully oxidize before being treated with heat. The longer oxidation process is what allows black teas to develop their pronounced classic black tea flavor.

Pu-erh — Pu-erh tea is fully oxidized and aged on top of that, producing a tea that will be super deep in color and aroma, reminiscent of a forest floor in a state of decomposition. While aging, this tea is contained in a tempered, humid environment in which microflora can flourish. This tea is often praised for its detoxifiction properties, earning it a side reputation as a classic hangover cure.

Tea plants can be harvested several times throughout the year. The tea harvest begins in spring, and can last from a few weeks to a few months, depending on the region and climate. Tea shrubs can be productive for many years, and in fact, some of the most prized teas come from ancient tea trees. The first (early spring) "flush" or plucking is awaited with great anticipation. Tea is an agricultural product, and growing conditions vary year to year. The complexity of taste, the variety of types and the seemingly unending ways to savor tea make it intriguing and exciting. Just as it is with different wine vintages, a favorite tea one year may not thrill you the next year—or it just might completely blow your socks off!

THE CHEMISTRY OF THE LEAF

What's in this leaf that makes it so special? And why is it so powerful? We need to get the chemistry down, because there's a lot of complex stuff going on in the tea leaf. Tea is made up of thousands of different molecules. What's going on in a live *Camellia sinensis* leaf changes as that leaf is processed into a finished tea product. During the processing of the tea leaf, many chemicals are broken down and transformed into new molecules. Then there's the question of what actually infuses into your cup. Over 99 percent of what's in your tea beverage is just plain water. Extracted molecules from the tea leaf make up only one-third of one percent of your brew, so we need to take a really close look at the tea solids that are able to make their way into your cup during the infusion process. All of the molecules featured in the diagram on page 31 extract in both hot and cold water, so they can make their way into your beverage however you choose to brew your tea leaves. Spoiler alert: There's good news for you ahead.

The following molecules are all naturally occurring plant substances called phytochemicals (*phyto* means "plant" in Greek). Phytochemicals encompass thousands of different compounds, many of them having unique benefits. Collectively, these nutrients are thought to be what gives plant-based foods and beverages their disease-fighting powers. Tea's antioxidants are phytochemicals.

POLYPHENOLS

The type of phytochemicals which are most plentiful in your tea are the very same ones that fire up the enzymes involved in immune response—polyphenol antioxidants. They make up a full 40 percent of the active ingredients in your cup of tea. These kick-ass, immune system–boosters do a great job getting through the whole tea-making process and then infusing their way into your tea cup. What's more, all teas contain a variety of these tea polyphenols, although their mix varies, depending on the type of tea. That's because the chemical composition of various teas differ as a result of how they're produced. It's during the longer oxidation period that some simple polyphenols are converted to larger, longer polyphenol molecules. These bigger molecules are what give black tea its darker, reddish color. Tea polyphenols are among the most efficient of all free radical scavengers, and they're more readily absorbed than most other antioxidants found in plant-based foods and beverages.

Flavonoids

You'll often hear the terms "polyphenols" and "flavonoids" used interchangeably, although flavonoids are actually just one type of polyphenol compound. There are more than 6,000 types of flavonoids, and they're a very diverse group. When people recommend that you eat all the colors of the rainbow, that's because they want you to get the beneficial flavonoid phytonutrients, which give almost all fruits and vegetables their vivid colors.

Flavanols

A yummy subset of flavonoids are flavanols, prevalent in tea, cocoa and red wine. These antioxidants have been studied extensively in humans in relation to heart health and brain function, as well as disease prevention. The FDA has not approved any health claim or approved any as pharmaceutical drugs.

Catechins

Within the flavanol family, the tea polyphenols which get top billing are the catechins (kat-eh-kins), and tea is the best source of catechins in the human diet. Catechins are particularly active flavanols and super potent antioxidants in free radical scavenging.

EGCg

The most dynamic of the catechins is epigallocatechin gallate (EGCg). EGCg is the darling of tea polyphenols with good reason. Studies have shown that its antioxidant capacity is 100 times more powerful than vitamin C in protecting DNA from damage by free radicals. Its also been shown to be twice as powerful as resveratrol, the key antioxidant in red wine. Although there are many different types of beneficial compounds in tea, current research indicates that EGCg is the polyphenol antioxidant with the broadest and most potent ability to protect your body's cells from cancer.

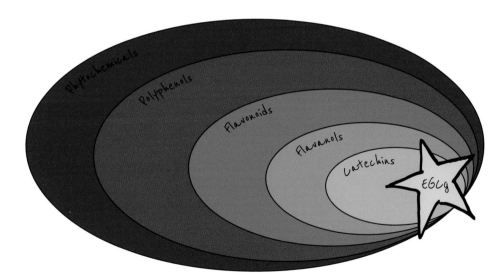

Polyphenols are the strongest biologically active agents in tea, but there are other fun tea molecules in your cup as well. Two of those key players are caffeine and theanine.

Caffeine

Say hello. Caffeine is the best known molecule in tea, and the most prized over the ages. People crave it—you might have a love/hate relationship with it. It increases perceived energy levels as well as cognitive ability, and it's one of the most studied ingredients in the plant world. Tea leaves contain about 2 to 5 percent caffeine by weight. Different steeping recommendations for different types of tea means that each cup will vary in caffeine levels. The longer you steep your tea, the more caffeine you'll get in your cup. It's also important to note that the effects of caffeine in tea are often reported as being different than the effects of caffeine from coffee. This is thought to be due to an amino acid unique to tea: theanine.

Theanine

L-Theanine, also simply known as theanine (thee-ah-neen), is the feel-good active ingredient in tea. Together with caffeine, as it occurs naturally in tea, it can produce a calm, yet focused state of mind. This amino acid is psychoactive, which means that it crosses your blood-brain barrier and goes to work in your head. Specifically, theanine increases alpha brain wave activity, which helps to relax the mind without inducing drowsiness, creating a state of deep relaxation in combination with mental alertness. Research has indicated that theanine can improve the speed, performance and accuracy in demanding tasks requiring cognition. (Translation: It will make you more productive at school or at work.) It's also thought to reduce attention deficit hyperactivity disorder (ADHD) hyperactivity and is used as a natural alternative to ADHD prescriptions.

MEDICINE OR BEVERAGE?

Tea is a plant-based beverage. When you steep tea, you're extracting its powerful nutrients. They work like a healing blanket for your body's cells, nourishing them and shutting down active agents and precursors of disease, whether you're healthy or ailing. Despite its amazing healing power, most of us only begin to learn about tea's significant effects on our bodies when we're already faced with disease. Green tea is on a serious marketing high and you can find it at or near the top of any superfoods list. Let's get another thing straight: This isn't just a passing fad. People have been turning to this ancient elixir as a healthy beverage for almost 5,000 years and treatises on its health benefits have been written for over 1,000 years. Now, thanks to modern science, we have many medical studies to further illuminate these benefits. Americans have one of the highest rates of cancer incidence on the globe. Population studies have shown that cultures that are heavy tea drinkers have far lower cancer rates than Westerners. In particular, studies of human diets have linked populations who drink large amounts of green tea with lower risk for breast, ovarian, prostate, bladder, colon, pancreatic and esophageal cancers. Tea is the second most consumed beverage worldwide, behind water; but only sixth on the list in the U.S. behind water, soda, beer, milk and coffee. Part of the reason for tea's global appeal is cost-effectiveness, but the irony for those populations who can't afford bottled drinks is that the pure tea they're drinking is much better for them.

WHAT'S IN YOUR CUP?

Your cup of tea is 99 2/3% water & 1/3% tea solids.

Here's what you get in a single serving of tea made with 2 g of tea leaves:

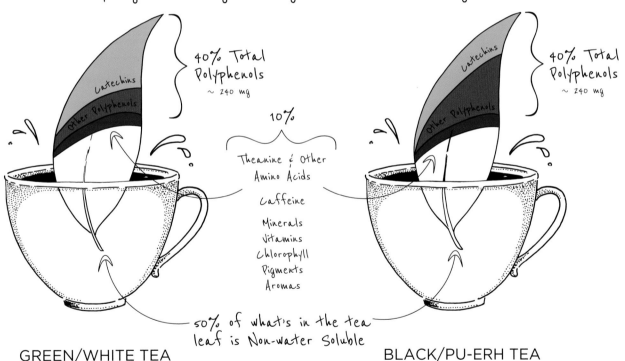

40% Total Polyphenols
~ 240 mg

Catechins

Other Polyphenols

10%

Theanine & Other Amino Acids

Caffeine

Minerals
Vitamins
Chlorophyll
Pigments
Aromas

40% Total Polyphenols
~ 240 mg

Catechins

Other Polyphenols

50% of what's in the tea leaf is Non-water Soluble

GREEN/WHITE TEA

BLACK/PU-ERH TEA

The concept of disease prevention by use of plant-based foods (and beverages such as tea) has been studied as a practical approach for thousands of years. In fact, tea's legacy began as one of a healthful beverage. Its historical beginnings in China date from 2737 BC, when the Chinese emperor Shen Nung, granddaddy of modern agriculture, is credited with its discovery. He was responsible for encouraging his people, who were suffering from the plague, to start boiling water before drinking it. The legend goes that the emperor was boiling a vat of water near a *Camellia sinensis* plant, and when a leaf floated in and infused the water, it produced an enchanting elixir that left the emperor feeling refreshed when he sipped the beverage. Thus tea was born. It's likely that tea was probably considered a medicinal beverage for the first few thousand years, and likely consumed like a vegetable in soup mixed with other ingredients such as salt, onions, orange peel and ginger.

If you look at dietary polyphenols consumed by all humans around the globe, tea is the number one source. Each cup of freshly brewed whole leaf tea can serve up over 200 mg of polyphenol antioxidants. By contrast, a serving of kale has about one-third as many and a serving of berries approximately one-half. Tea also shows higher antioxidant activities against free radicals than spinach, garlic and Brussels sprouts. Another point to keep in mind when comparing the antioxidant capacity of different foods and beverages is that it takes just a couple of grams of loose leaf tea to brew one cup. Gram for gram and penny for penny, tea is in the antioxidants bargain bin.

The benefits of having tea in your system manifest themselves in a myriad of ways. Tea helps to manage free radicals. (Think inflammation, stress and even signs of aging in skin.) It also has antibacterial properties, helping to protect your body from bacterial agents entering your body. (Think bad breath and stomach disorders.) Tea polyphenols damage the structure of microbes by attacking their cell membranes and by inhibiting bacterial enzymes essential to their growth. Drinking tea is a cost-effective way to detox, and yes, it works great as a hangover cure (especially pu-erh tea). Tea has also been shown to be an effective weapon in humans in the fight against cholesterol and high blood pressure. Studies also have shown that tea polyphenols could inhibit the onset and severity of arthritis in humans. Tea has even been shown to be effective against allergic reactions, as EGCg has been shown to block a key biochemical process in allergic responses. Tea is also known as the secret of the skinny—but thin can't compete with healthy!

CANCER HATES TEA

When cancer's winning against you, it succeeds in getting its rogue cells to multiply wildly out of control, triggers inflammation inside you and works to plunder your organism for blood vessels to fuel its tumor's growth. It stays 100 percent focused on wreaking havoc on your system in its glorious killer plan for metastasis to other organs in your body. The antioxidants in tea work like multitasking fiends to bash cancer during every stage in its attempted coup. Here are three ways tea can help you in the battle:

1. Research studies show tea polyphenols as being highly effective free radical scavengers. This puts the brakes on chemical mechanisms of oxidative stress. A whopping 40 percent of the active compounds in your tea are polyphenol antioxidants, whose action provides an additional layer of protection for your cells and molecules. This layer mitigates the possibility of abnormal cell growth caused by damage to your cellular DNA. Tea helps keep your first line of defense—your immune system—buzzing. **The best way to piss off cancer is to never even let it get a foothold against you.**

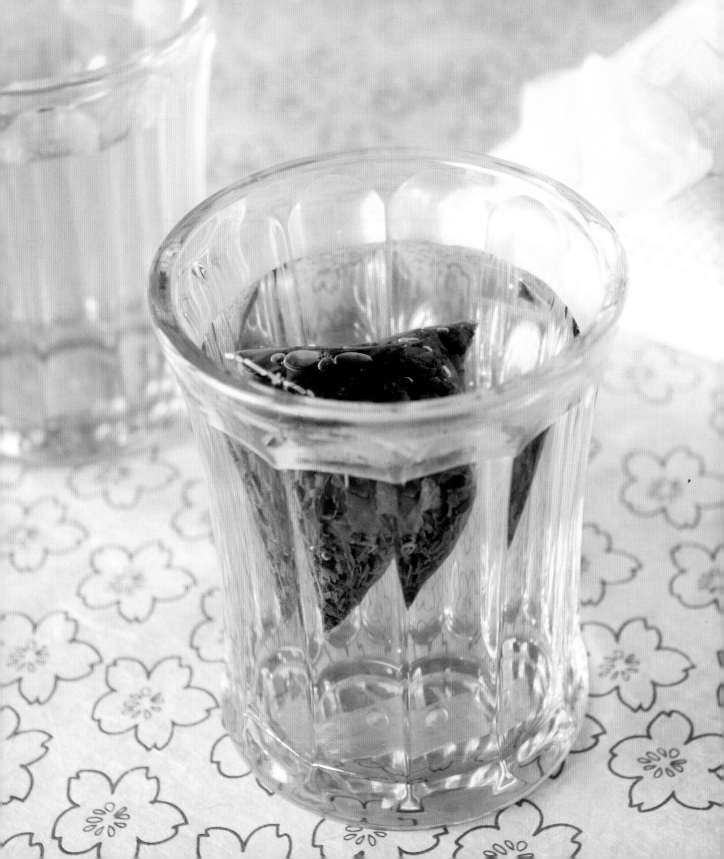

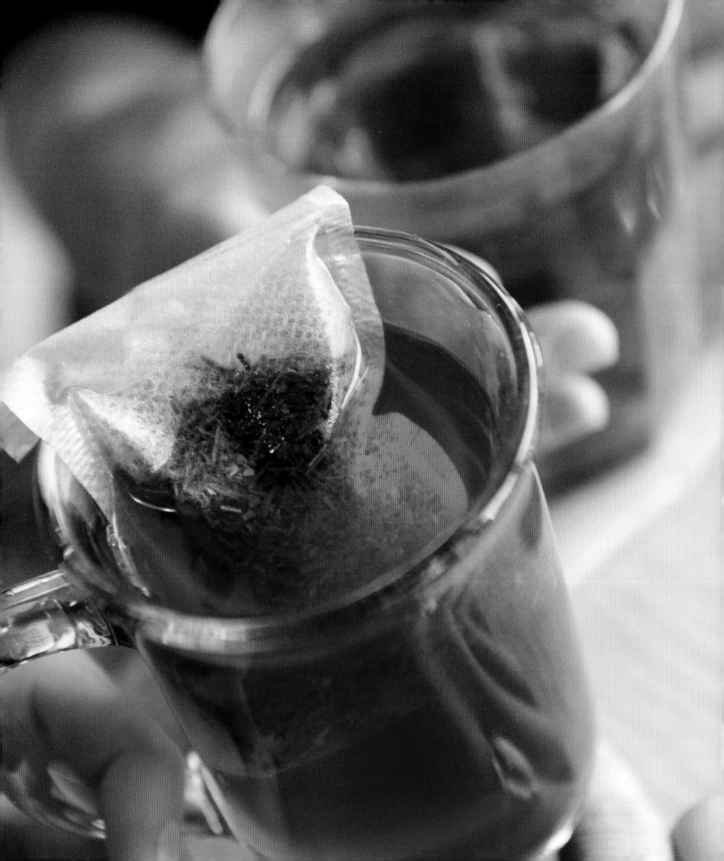

2. The proliferation of cancer requires enlisting your body's assistance to build a network of blood vessels, which becomes the tumor's mainline for oxygen and nutrients. Your body can actually get tricked into responding to these signals positively, not realizing the tumor growth is out to destroy it. If your body refuses to build these energy resources, cancerous cells die from lack of oxygen and nutrients, and the malignancy simply can't progress. Cancer cells need to be able to send signals to one another, as well as trickster messages to call your body for help to keep it growing. Tea fights cancer in this stage of progression by enlisting EGCg to inhibit the signaling—a very excellent tool in cancer defense.

3. To become a full-fledged malignancy, cancer cells need to achieve their goal of spreading to other organs in your body. To get this going, cancer needs to totally abolish your body's plan for natural cell death. Recent studies have indicated that tea catechins assist in the molecular mechanisms that regulate cell death, which is crucial in the regression of cancer in humans. The science suggests that tea polyphenols can work as anti-tumor agents by derailing cancer from its grand plan for limitless growth in your body.

Cancer treatment is a serious test. Cancer is a challenging disease to treat because the selective killing of tumor cells without harming too many healthy cells or the immune system is incredibly complicated. Annihilating all the malignant cells without actually killing the patient in the process sometimes requires therapies which feel like a chemical sledgehammer in the hands of a Neanderthal with bad aim. Cancer treatments being developed today employ selective targeting techniques, focusing on specifically attacking only cancer cells and their biochemical mechanisms. Their goal is to inhibit these processes, while minimizing harm to normal cells.

Tea polyphenols work in much the same way. They target many of the same specific cancer growth mechanisms. The therapeutic effectiveness of tea is in inhibiting the genesis, development and proliferation of cancers. There are studies that conclude positive health benefits of drinking tea against cancer progression, as well as studies that are inconclusive or show no benefits. The results are mixed. But taken in ensemble, the evidence weighs in strongly on the positive side for tea's antioxidant, anti-cancer benefits. **Tea alone will not cure or prevent cancer.** But everyone should know about the benefits of drinking tea. Steep like mad. Drink like your life depends on it. This small change to your every day can make a big difference. And cancer will just hate it.

-PART TWO-

DRINK UP
TO STARE
CANCER DOWN

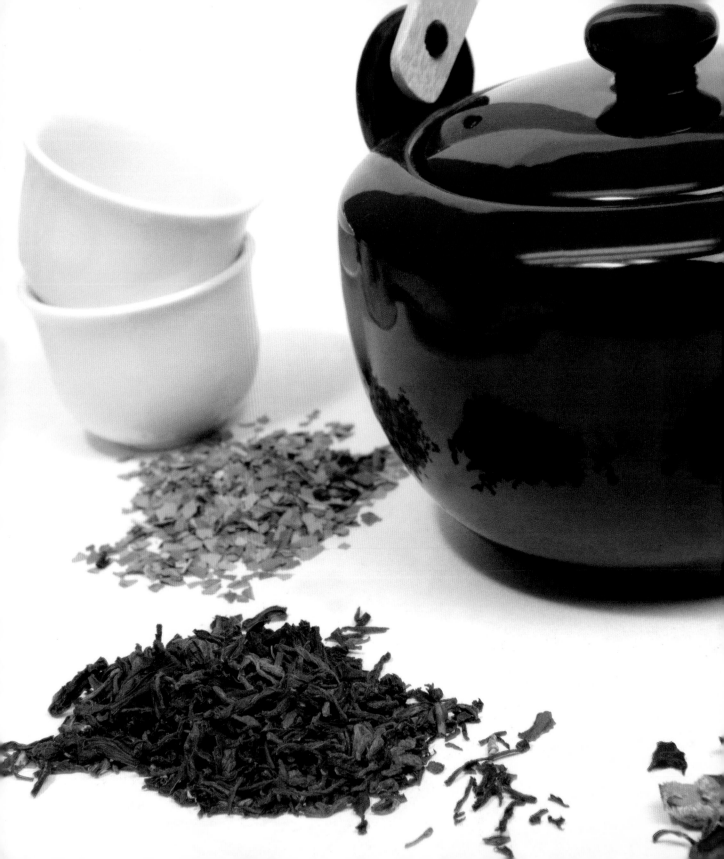

Chapter 2

STEEP YOUR OWN DAMN TEA

STEEP OR STEEP NOT. THERE IS NO TRY.

How I Learned to Love the Leaf: My Own Tea Story

As I was recovering from harsh cancer treatments, I started my research on preventative measures that I could take under my own control. The study that turned me on to tea, and in particular green tea, was one in which the results suggested the possibility that regular green tea consumption, of 3 to 5 cups (720 ml to 1.2 L) per day, may be preventive against the recurrence of cancer. The women who drank more than 3 cups (720 ml) per day experienced 57 percent fewer relapses of breast cancer than those who drank only 1 cup (240 ml) per day. There was sufficient statistical significance, and the study was on a large enough sample (5,264 person-years of follow-up) to compel me seek out Japanese whole leaf teas. I wanted the exact same thing these women were drinking. In a study of men with prostate cancer from the same time frame, it was found that drinking 5 cups (1.2 L) a day reduced the chance of tumor progression to an advanced stage by 50 percent.

Before that, even though I was a tea lover, and a pretty regular tea drinker (though not multiple servings a day, regularly), I had only ever enjoyed black tea. I think I'd tried green tea a few times and it really didn't sit well with me. Drinking green tea daily was a self-imposed acquired habit, one which took me years to truly enjoy and look forward to. For me, the better quality green teas, such as the finer-leafed teas or ceremony-grade matcha, were easier to get down than the bigger leaf, bigger stem teas, but it was still like taking medicine for quite a while. As I researched tea chemistry and the tea and cancer medical studies further, I learned that black teas yield legitimately awesome active substances as well. I happily balanced out my tea drinking rituals with lots of my personal faves, such as Earl Grey, Assam breakfast teas and Keemun. Today, I'm actually joyful when I reach for Japanese green tea first in the morning, because it's what my body and taste buds are craving, and it no longer feels like an obligatory kind of health insurance.

IMPOSTER TEA?

It's easy to take in the billboard ads, drink the green tea Kool-Aid and get seduced into thinking "This stuff's good for me!" Like millions of people every day, you may think you're doing your body good by grabbing that bottle of tea at the convenience store. But read the label, and you'll likely find it's filled with tons of laboratory manufactured chemicals with no connections to the plant kingdom. The actual tea and polyphenol content in most of those canned and bottled teas is merely a trace. All those benefits you got excited about in the first chapter? They only apply to freshly steeped whole leaf tea. So, feeling robbed? If you want the whole cookie instead of the crumbs off the factory floor, it's simple—steep your own damn tea. Now let's take a look at the many reasons why.

JUST GIVE ME THE NUMBER

The USDA Database for the Flavonoid Content of Selected Foods is one of many sources that sheds some light on fresh brewed versus bottled. This hefty report, updated every few years, provides measurements of various polyphenol levels for hundreds of food items. It includes some brewed teas, as well as ready-to-drink (RTD) bottled teas. What it tells us is that EGCg values for a single serving of **freshly brewed green teas range from five to twenty times higher** than the measured EGCg value in RTD green tea. Would you have ever thought that your $2 to $3 bottle of green tea could provide less than a tenth the EGCg of the cup of tea you brew at home for less than 20 cents?

The next time you're pushing a shopping cart full of tea products around the grocery store, take a closer look at the labels. Do they say anything about the actual antioxidant content, or are you just buying tea flavor? My colleagues and I went through a multitude of grocery stores and photographed labels on every tea product we could get our hands on. Our experience showed that although about one-third of them reported caffeine content, fewer than one in twenty addressed antioxidant content at all. It should probably be illegal for some of these drinks to actually call themselves tea.

What's more, the added sugars in RTD tea products are often as bad as what you get in a carbonated beverage or a candy bar. It's no surprise that Americans consume about one-fifth of our calories from things we drink. Sugary teas are among the worst offenders, alongside soft drinks, energy drinks, fruit drinks and coffee drinks. Heck, iced tea and sweet tea were invented here! In fact, it happened at the 1904 World's Fair in St. Louis. A group of tea producers from India had set up a fancy booth to promote their black teas, but the sweltering summer heat and humidity prompted them to serve the tea over ice, just to get people to try it. In the 100 years since then, consumption of iced tea in the U.S. has grown to over 40 billion cups (10 million L) per year, and the vast majority of it is heavily sweetened and flavored. It now accounts for 80 percent of the tea consumed in the U.S. This evolution has helped develop a tea habit to where it comes laden with sugar and super weak in antioxidants.

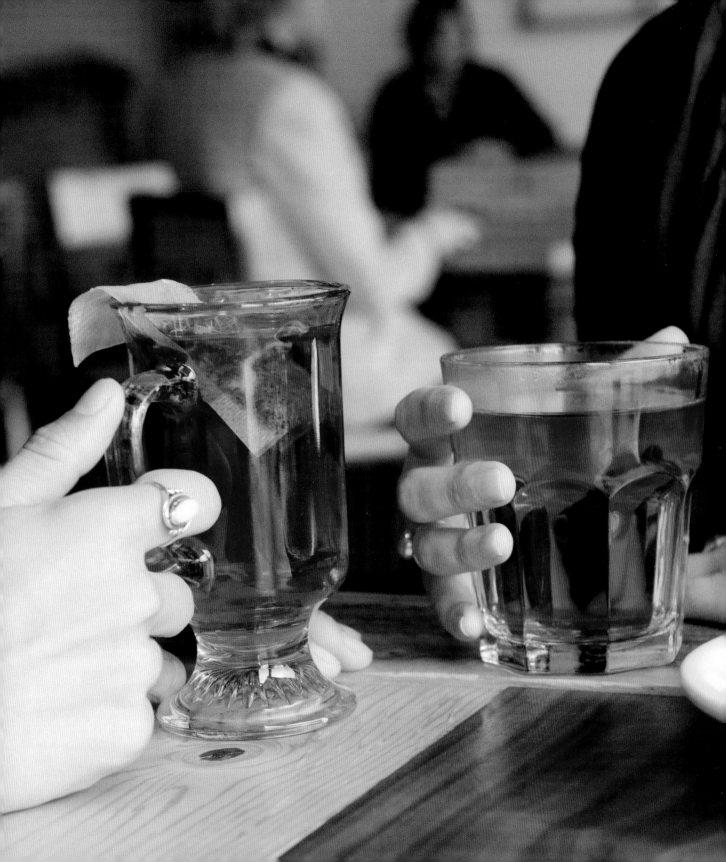

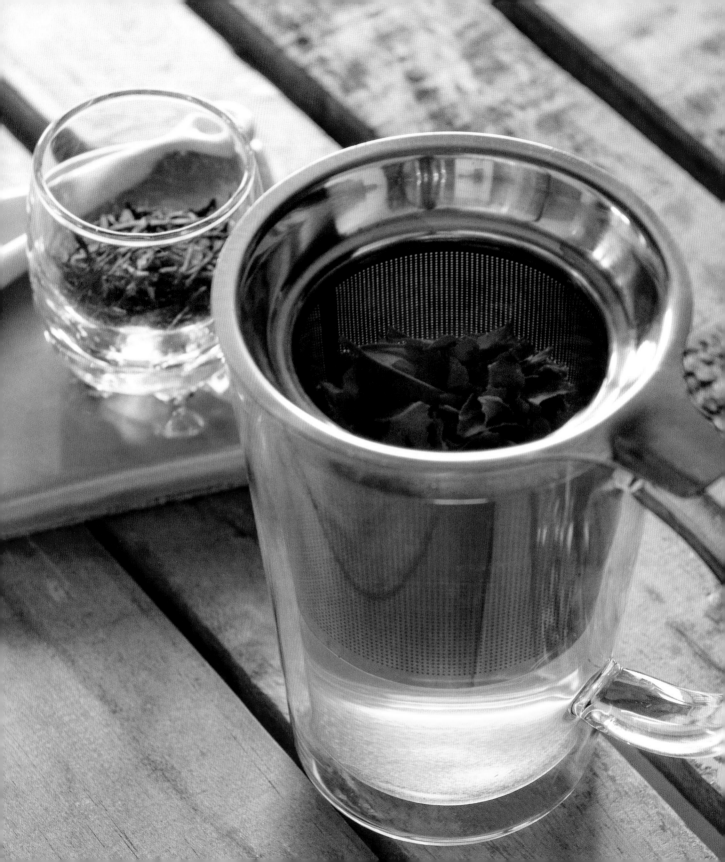

ABOUT GREEN TEA

Green tea is to black as flute is to cello or spring morning is to winter night. Green tea leaves picked in the morning can be processed and ready to be brewed that very same night. Shortly after they're picked from the plant, the leaves are dried out by heating them in ovens, pans over fire or with steam. This removes almost all of the moisture in the tea leaves and arrests the natural oxidation process, inhibiting any further chemical or color change. This bypass of an extended oxidation period is what allows green tea to retain most of its natural bright-green color, simple polyphenols, vitamin C, amino acids and plant-like aromas. The taste of green tea is therefore more fresh and subtle than the more oxidized oolong or black teas. Its caffeine effect is of a nearly steady, mild high with no big peaks or plunges. This is thanks to theanine, the alpha brain activity-enhancing amino acid, found in high concentrations in green tea. With its growing reputation as a powerful natural source of antioxidants, green tea is widely used as a natural active ingredient in food and cosmetics. The list of touted health benefits in these products may range from fighting aging and disease to weight loss, all of which work to further promote its popularity.

Tasting and selecting teas is a subject matter that takes years of experience and training of the palate. There are five main characteristics on which tea leaves are appraised. These include the appearance of the leaf both before and after steeping, the color of the infusion and the resulting tea's aroma and taste. Green tea leaves come in a wide range of colors, shapes and sizes, which are dictated by their origin and processing. China and Japan are traditionally where green teas were cultivated, although today you can also find green teas from many countries, including Korea, Vietnam, Sri Lanka and India. There's even a tea plantation that produces green tea just outside Charleston, SC in the U.S. and small, budding tea farms in Hawaii, the Bay Area and Canada. The methods by which green teas are grown, harvested and processed vary wildly from region to region. For the most part, Chinese green teas grow in the full sun. The names of Chinese teas denote leaf styles and often make reference to the region where the tea is produced. They include such classics as dragonwell and gunpowder, as well as many teas with poetic names such as clouds and mist. Some Japanese green teas spend part of their growing season in the shade, which increases the chlorophyll content in the leaves and gives them a deeper green color. Japanese-style tea leaves also tend to be finer and thinner at the conclusion of their processing. The names of Japanese teas generally end in -cha (meaning "tea"), for example, sencha, bancha, hojicha, genmaicha and matcha.

NOT ALL TEAS ARE CREATED EQUAL

The best reason for steeping your own tea, or at least the one that will get you the most immediate gratification, is that a fresh steeped mug of whole leaf tea tastes infinitely better than something from a bottle or a flat, wimpy tea bag. Most people grow up thinking tea totally lacks in taste—kind of like the stale biscuits you'd imagine old ladies dunking in their tea. That's not totally without foundation since most of the tea available to us in grocery stores and restaurants today is actually pretty tasteless, thanks to the amazing invention of the tea bag. Sadly, the tea that is readily available in the U.S. is, for the most part, little more than low-end tea. It's geared more toward efficiency and convenience than quality. Although the debate generally pits loose leaf tea against tea bags, it really should come down to a question of the quality of the leaf. Most tea bags are stuffed with the lowest grades of tea. Those grades are technically referred to as dust and fannings. **Are you drinking a whole leaf tea, or is that tea dust you're steeping?** Tea bags use this dust because no one can really see what's inside the paper filter. Low-grade tea helps get to the target price point of most tea bags, and tea dust infuses faster than a full leaf. It's also easier to run tiny bits of tea leaf through a tea bagging machine than fluffy, full leaf tea. Studies have shown that tea prepared using tea bags has lower antioxidant capacity than full leaf tea. The same dusty bits which make tea bags tea less effective from a health standpoint also make it less aromatic, less tasty and less pretty. So let's just set a rule right now: no flat tea bags.

If you suffer separation anxiety about leaving your trusted tea bags, consider this: A box of 20 typical tea bags in the supermarket costs about $3.99. These are usually blended with up to 60 varieties of the pathetic lowest grade remains of the vibrant tea leaf and will run you about 20 cents per cup. If you compare the value of the tea bag's per-pound (500 g) cost of over $100 per pound (500 g), you could instead get a premier loose leaf tea, with its full-size, hand-picked and beautifully processed leaves which will yield about 200 cups (40 L) per pound (450 g). You'll be drinking a tea that is the equivalent of a Chateau Lafite-Rothschild wine. The better whole leaf teas will also yield more cups of tea than the mediocre ones, and, quite ironically, don't cost much more. Also consider how the quality of your leaf and resulting beverage affects the amount of tea polyphenols you're getting from every serving of your tea.

The tea bag was invented accidently in the early 20th century by a tea merchant in New York. He'd been sending out small samples of his tea in little silk bags, and even though he didn't intend it as such, his clients started using the sample bags as silken infusers, dumping the whole thing in the teapot. He actually got complaints about the product before it was even born. People wanted the mesh bags to be more open in the weave of the material, so the water could flow in and out more readily for better infusion. The smart tea merchant rolled with this, the trend caught on and within 10 years there were tea bag manufacturing machines making paper filter bags of a similar type to the ones which are prevalent in the market today. Tea bags account for more than 90 percent of today's tea market in the U.S., Canada and the U.K.—where they were only introduced after World War II. The Brits initially stuck their noses up at this American invention that offered lower grade tea in a bag and had no intention of giving up their full leaf infusions. But ultimately, convenience won out over tradition. Like many time-saving household gadgets of the 1950s, the tea bag gained popularity on the grounds that it eliminated the need to empty out spent tea leaves from the teapot. Thus, even one of the world's strongest tea cultures got over the appearance and quality shortcomings of the humble tea bag.

DID YOU GET AN ANTIOXIDANT BANG FOR YOUR BUCK?

	READY-TO-DRINK TEA	GROCERY TEA BAGS	PREMIUM TEA SACHETS	LOOSE WHOLE LEAF TEA
	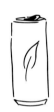	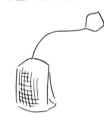	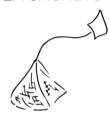	
$/SERVING	$0.50-$3.00	$0.10-$0.20	$0.30-$2.00	$0.10-$1.00
TIME TO PREPARE	-0-	2-3 minutes	2-5 minutes	2-5 minutes
		← + time to heat water →		
POLYPHENOLS PER SERVING	Trace	Trace-Medium	High-Very High	High-Very High
BANG FOR YOUR ANTIOXIDANT $	Poor	Poor-Good	Good-Great	Great-off-the-charts

Note: Not all tea bags are created equal. Larger, three-dimensional tea bags made from mesh fabric are not new. In fact, that's how they started out. Fast forward 100 years, and the recent trend for higher-end premium teas is to go back in the direction of the early silken sachets. These newer three-dimensional tea sachets offer a more open weave material than a paper filter does, and more volume, which can accommodate full leaf teas. Many of these bigger mesh bags are filled with the same quality of loose leaf tea you find in tea tins and in bulk. What you'll drink is very much the same as a freshly steeped loose leaf tea, only without needing to use an infuser. These are super convenient, though more pricey, of course, than steeping your tea loose. With the added convenience you also lose the flexibility of how much tea you get to put into your mug.

ALL THE TEAS IN CHINA

You'd be hard pressed to find a tea bag in China nor can you get through a business meeting in that country without being served tea. And I don't just mean *tea* business meetings—we're talking *any* kind of meeting. As the largest producers of tea in the world, the Chinese are so very proud of their product, and in a most localized way because the diversity of regional tea choices in China is as colorful as it is for cheese and wine in France. Every region, and in some tea-intense areas, every village has their unique tea and methods of producing tea, and of course they're all very excited to get you to agree that theirs is the very best around.

The Chinese tea ceremony, called *Gongfu Cha*, is the complete antithesis to grab and go. The meaning of Gongfu (or *Kungfu*, as it's known in the martial arts) is "skill achieved through hard work and practice," and *Cha* is the Chinese word for tea. Its intention is to produce a drink that is satisfying to the soul. Many Chinese people can go through this many-steps many-motions tea service while multitasking, without ever skipping a beat in the business conversation. Traditionally, large-leafed teas are placed in very small porcelain or clay teapots, or lidded cups, and then they are rinsed and infused with hot water—repeatedly. The tea is served in tiny cups less than an ounce (30 ml) in capacity, and the tea that's served is treated and tastes like a precious elixir.

The majority of teas that get served in China are not available for export. The Gongfu tea ceremony process goes on and on, for at least five infusions, and sometimes many more, using the same leaves in the tiny steeping vessel. Oftentimes, ceramic tea pets adorn the tea tray on which this spectacle takes place. Every tea and every ceremony in China creates a unique visual and taste memory, and I can say from experience that it almost always succeeds in meeting its traditional goal of satisfying the soul.

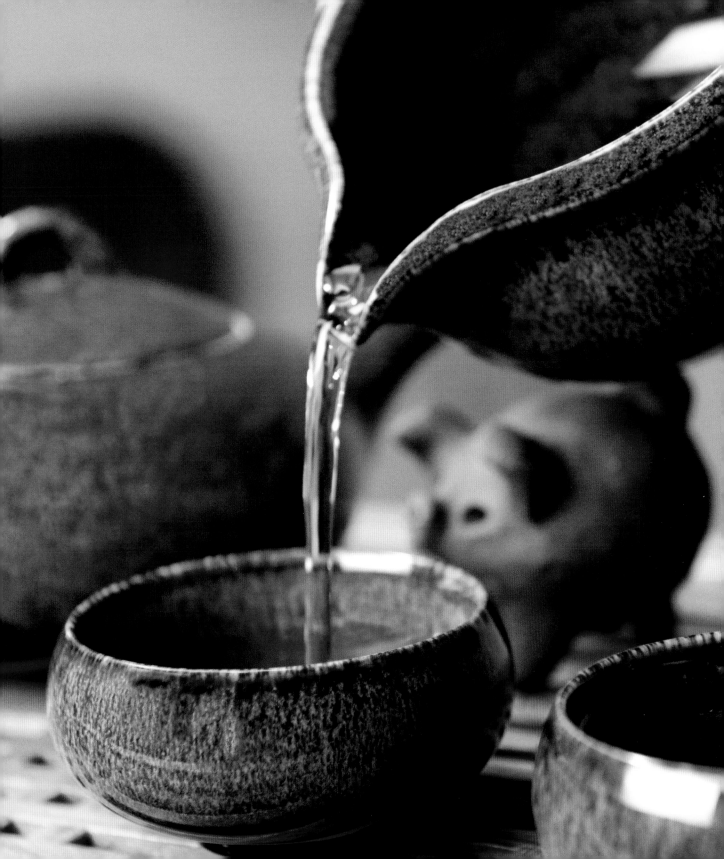

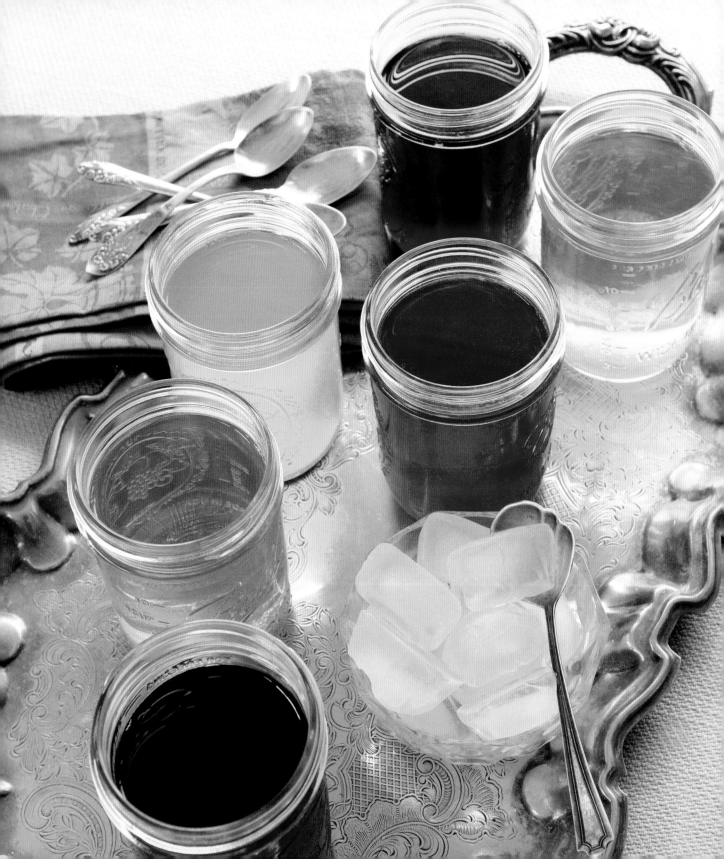

REAL TEA = REAL BENEFITS

Beyond the distinction between leaves and dust, the quantity of polyphenols in your tea will vary depending on tea type, freshness, growing region, tea plant cultivar, the season of harvest and how it's processed. **As far as total antioxidants go, all quality whole leaf teas are pretty comparable.** Green teas are higher in catechin polyphenols, and black teas are higher in the more complex tea polyphenols. Photosynthesis produces sugars, which in turn produce polyphenols. This means that teas grown in sunshine can exhibit higher levels of antioxidants than the same tea plants grown in shade. It's true that there will be some variation in the type and level of antioxidants based on all the above factors, but if you steep a cup of quality whole leaf tea for yourself, you're bound to be getting a rich dose of beneficial phytochemicals. About 30 percent of the tea leaves infuse into your beverage as tea solids, and about 40 percent of those solids will be polyphenols. **A serving of tea made with 1.5 tsp (2 g) tea leaves will yield over 200 mg of tea polyphenols in each serving.**

The dictionary says: "Steep: to put (something) in a liquid for a period of time." According to Merriam-Webster, "steep suggests either the extraction of an essence (as of tea leaves) by the liquid or the imparting of a quality (as a color) to the thing immersed. First known use: 1555." When you're steeping loose leaf tea, you're just putting water in contact with dried tea leaves. That's a whole lot less complicated than you might expect. Steeping from fine handpicked leaves takes just a little more effort than dunking a tea bag, as well as a few seconds more time.

Steeping your own makes even the high-end healthiest and tastiest teas a bargain. Yup, loose-leaf tea is a screaming deal, which seems to be a well-protected secret. Who knows, you might even learn to enjoy those extra couple of minutes it takes to watch the leaves unfurl and infuse to their full flavor and aroma.

If your head feels like it's spinning with numbers and options, don't despair: **Just steep real tea leaves that look like they come from a real plant.** Follow that one step and believe me, this won't be your grandma's tea party. Once a tea drinker graduates from a low-end tea bag to whole leaf teas, he or she is on their way to a whole new world. The choices of available loose leaf teas can stagger the imagination. Do you still have some lame tea bags laying around? Don't fret: Save the little tea bags to get rid of the circles under your eyes when you're tired. If nothing else, cool, damp tea bags are really great for that!

ABOUT STEEPING TEA

It's one thing to have killer catechins in a fresh tea leaf. Getting these to effectively infuse into your tea beverage and work on your cells is quite another story. Recall that the fraction of actual tea solids in your cup is one-third of one percent, the rest being water. Quality matters. If you've never had loose leaf tea (which is true for most people in this country) you're in for a mind-blowing treat. Since I've been working in the tea industry, I've had the honor of serving many people their first cup of loose leaf tea, and in fact, it's one of my favorite things to do. You wouldn't believe the fun eye-opening expressions and little smiles on people's faces after their first sip of freshly infused goodness.

Tea Leaves + Hot Water + Time = Tea. That's it! Don't let yourself be intimidated.

Water is clutch.
It makes up 99.6 percent of your tea. Use cold water fresh from the tap. If you don't like your tap water, filtered or purified water is great, but distilled water is not because it'll make your tea taste flat.

Watch temperature, timing and proportions—think baking.
You'll figure out exactly how much tea and water to use, and how long you like it steeped, but start with one rounded teaspoon (about 2 g) of leaves per 8 ounces (240 ml) water. It's rare to make a new tea perfectly to your taste on the first try, but do try starting with your tea's recommended amount (Chapter 9, page 143). Tea polyphenols infuse rapidly, so you don't need to over-steep your tea to get the good stuff.

Repeat.
Many whole leaf teas can be re-infused. The same leaves can be steeped over and over again, and yes, you'll continue to get some health benefits out of those leaves for as long as they continue to infuse flavor and color.

Drink it fresh.
That means today. Tea will stay fresh and potent for about 24 hours after it's steeped. Drink it while it's still fresh and brimming with serious active ingredients.

Hold the milk and sugar.
Adding milk can blunt the favorable effects of tea on your arteries, and sugar is an agent for inflammation.

Add lemon, if you like.
Research has shown that adding ascorbic acid helps to preserve the polyphenols in tea, thus increasing their ability to be absorbed by the body.

Try a cold brew.

Did you know that you could sip fresh tea all day long without ever using a kettle? Cold brewing tea is easy-peasy and for many teas yields a most amazing brew. When you bring your dried tea leaves in contact with hot or boiling water, they infuse much faster, but this process also transforms some of the active ingredients as it extracts them. The slower process of steeping in cold water results in a simpler and purer extraction than when you steep your tea hot. A cold-brewed tea's flavor is somewhat different than the hot-brew version. It's usually smoother and cleaner. Cold-brew tea isn't just for the brainless, it can actually be better for you as it yields similar, and in some cases better, antioxidant levels than teas brewed hot. So stop making your iced tea with hot water.

Chill out.

Steeping tea will become second nature to you in no time. You'll learn to make a perfect-tasting, healthy mug of tea in less than five minutes, start to finish. Time is your most precious commodity, isn't it? Cancer doesn't respect your time, but a tea habit totally can.

Make it your own.

Steep what you love. Guaranteed, every time I give a talk on tea and health, one of the first questions is always "But which tea's the healthiest one for me to drink?" My recommendation is always the same: Drink the tea you love the most, because that's the one you'll drink the most of. Sure, they vary in terms of relative concentrations of specific polyphenols. But if you're drinking a catechin-rich green tea like it's medicine and can barely stomach it, how much of it will you really want to drink? If your palate goes crazy happy when you steep up a smoky breakfast tea, my take is—indulge yourself. You'll drink two mugs of that tea in the time it would take you to get through a fraction of a serving of a green tea you don't enjoy. All whole leaf teas you steep fresh are antioxidant-rich.

Don't let me or anyone else tell you what your tea should taste like. Make it as light or strong, cold or hot as you want. That's totally your choice. Just try to do yourself and your teeth a favor and learn to crave it without sugar. Once this ancient brew becomes part of your daily ritual, you'll know how you like it best. Mix it up. This not only makes your tea day more interesting, but can get your body exposed to a variety of polyphenols, each with their own unique biochemical mechanisms and benefits. There's such an amazing range of colors, flavors, aromas and caffeine levels in tea. **You'll likely come out ahead if you just indulge yourself with your favorite teas.**

Cold Brew Heaven

Nothing could be easier, and the results are—you got it—heavenly! You'll feel like you're floating above the clouds as you sip on this cold brew.

Yield: Two 8-ounce (240 ml) servings

16 oz (480 ml) coconut water

2 tsp (3 g) white or green tea leaves

Combine ingredients in water bottle or mason jar for 10 to 15 minutes. Strain out tea leaves, and enjoy a sip of heaven!

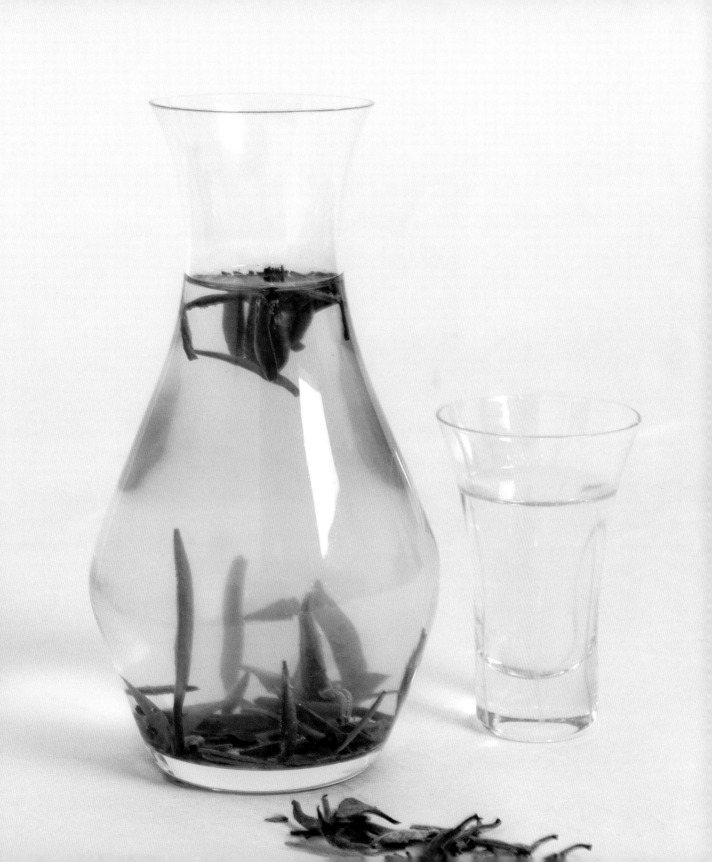

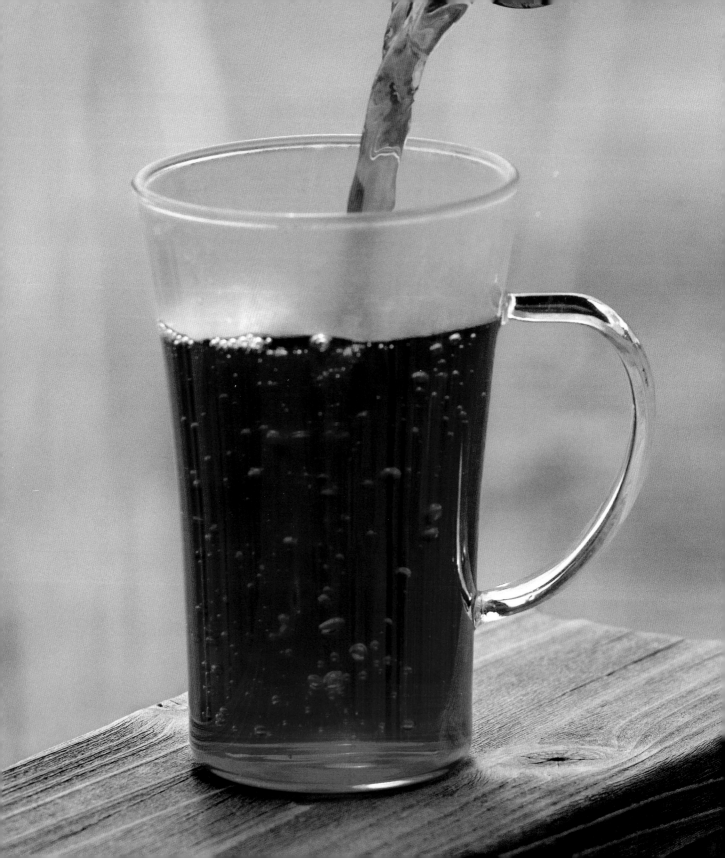

Chapter 3

DRINK LIKE YOUR LIFE DEPENDS ON IT

YOUR LIFE MATTERS

Cleveland Clinic Employee Wellness Program

The Cleveland Clinic, one of the world's most respected academic medical centers, is also a leader in implementing wellness programs that aggressively advocate healthy living.

Ten years ago, under the guidance of New York Times *best-selling author and wellness authority Dr. Michael Roizen, the hospital implemented an Employee Wellness Program. This program offers reduced health insurance premiums to employees who pass a positive health threshold. But the program doesn't exclude those who don't pass. They can also qualify for a premium discount if they choose to participate in a disease management program for their particular chronic condition that prevented them from passing the threshold. The program pays for employees to participate in activities ranging from Weight Watchers to tobacco treatment, and even offers yoga classes and a running club.*

When asked whether the program showed any quantifiable benefits, David Pauer, Director of Wellness for Employee Health at the Cleveland Clinic said, "Absolutely! Employee Wellness has saved about 85 million dollars in healthcare costs over the life of the program. We can feel confident in this estimate because the program was designed such that cost wouldn't be a barrier to the utilization of health services—employees have no deductibles and no co-insurance payments." In their dedication to helping their 90,000 employees achieve optimal well-being and a higher quality of life, the Cleveland Clinic is demonstrating the consequences of certain preventable conditions and their effects on the healthcare system.

"The biggest value of the program is in that it actually motivates people to do something about their health," asserts Pauer. "Employees can earn a 30 percent discount on premiums by participating, which for a family of four can add up to about $1,400 a year. Our activity device program is extremely popular. Only a certain population will join a fitness center, because it's limiting. Think about what it would be like if you had to have all your meals in one building. The activity device program motivates you to be active all the time, and people will actually do that to qualify for the discount." In addition, Pauer says that just offering a stimulus for program participants to get in and see the doctor for checkups has uncovered 50 to 60 cases of cancer which might otherwise have gone untreated far longer.

TEA HABITS BY THE NUMBERS

One: All teas come from 1 single plant species (*Camellia sinensis*).

Two: Tea is the 2nd most consumed beverage worldwide, behind water.

Three: Worldwide, people drink 3 times more tea than coffee, but in the U.S., people drink 3 times more coffee than tea.

Four: Basic tea types:
- Green/White (Not oxidized)
- Oolong (Partially Oxidized)
- Black (Fully Oxidized)
- Pu-erh (Oxidized and Aged)

Five: 5 cups (1.2 L) of fresh tea per day to get you into a routine that maximizes cancer prevention.

Six: Tea is the 6th most consumed beverage in the U.S., behind water, carbonated soft drinks, beer, milk and coffee.

Seven: In the top tea drinking nations the average tea drinkers use 7 pounds (3.2 kg) of tea leaves annually. In the U.S., the average is ½ pound (250 g) of tea leaves.

Eight: 80 billion servings of tea are consumed in the U.S. annually. The vast majority of these are iced, sweet tea and bottled. Only a tiny fraction is freshly steeped, as opposed to the rest of the world, who tend to steep their own tea.

Nine: The average amount of tea consumed annually per capita in the U.S. is 9 gallons (34 L). By contrast, the average number of gallons of carbonated soft drinks consumed annually in the U.S. is 45 gallons (170 L).

Ten: The number of different teas in the cupboard of a U.S. tea lover, on average, is 10.

Fifteen: A cup of high-end loose leaf tea you steep yourself costs about 15 cents.

BAD HABITS DIE HARD

Many population-based research studies inform us that cancer rates tend to be lower in countries where people regularly consume tea. On a global scale, we are tea dilettantes here in the U.S. The average American drinks the equivalent of just over a half pound (250 g) of tea per year. That barely breaks us into the top 35 tea-drinking nations. The top tea drinkers by comparison are countries which include the Middle East, North Africa, Turkey and the British Isles who consume the equivalent of nearly 7 pounds (3.2 kg) per person per year. Based on a standard serving of 1 teaspoon (about 2 g) of leaves, that amounts to an average of between four and five servings of tea every single day, compared with a person in the U.S. drinking just one serving every three days. We're a coffee-drinking nation, which if you examine beverage preferences worldwide, makes us an exception. In most countries, 3 cups (720 ml) of tea are drunk for every cup (240 ml) of coffee, whereas in this country, it's exactly the opposite. Tea is far more universal and it's not limited to exclusive segments of society. Rich or poor, warm climates or cold, in happy or sad times, **tea is the beverage that most people on this planet reach for**. After water, it's the second most consumed drink in the world. Billions of people start and often continue their days with this hot and stimulating beverage.

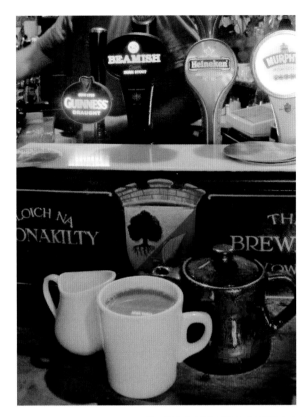

Tea drinking habits in the U.S. are beginning to change and evolve into some healthier choices. Tea is hot. Conversely, sodas are under scrutiny and trending downward and so is fruit juice. It's a dramatic time in the U.S. beverage industry, with the biggest carbonated soft drinks manufacturers expanding their product lines to highlight teas, all kinds of colors and flavors of waters and energy drinks. Regardless of how much sugar and caffeine they may contain, these are all boldly referred to as healthy beverages. There's a lot of hypocrisy and mislabeling here, and many of those wholesome-looking bottles and cans screaming TEA can barely qualify as either healthy or tea. Small batch and quality craft manufacture are also beverage categories on a rapid rise, especially in the alcoholic beverage space, and this will likely have a positive ripple effect in non-alcoholic single-serving drinks, hopefully leading to more quality selections in the future. Even as we start to move in the right direction, **as a nation we still drink about four times as much soda pop as we do tea**. Not a great endorsement for taking wellness into our own hands.

TIME FOR A CUPPA?

The Irish have a long-standing love affair with "tay," as they call it, out-drinking all their neighbors in the British Isles. The average tea consumption in Ireland per citizen is four to six cups per day—an excess of a quart (1 L) per day. It's quite the treat, as a tea lover, to be asked at least half a dozen times each day, "Time for a Cuppa?" (*Cupan Tae* in Gaelic). There's no need for cafés in a place chock-full of comfy, friendly pubs which open well before noon, when almost everyone's sitting at the bar with a pot of tea in front of them. Later in the afternoon, the stout starts pouring. Now how cool is that?

Unfortunately, there are no full leaves in sight (well over 90 percent of the teas are in bags), and I've yet to run into a green tea on the Emerald Isle. Assam, the largest tea-producing region in India, is who's supplying the base tea for these parts. It's the heartiest and most well known black tea. As the saying goes, "If strength is your weakness, Assam is your tea." Ever tried Irish Breakfast Tea? An absolute eye-opener tea, it's perfect for that first cup of the day. Strong and dark, it's served hot, with milk and sugar as options more often than not. I don't know if it's the tea, the gorgeous countryside or the amazing warmth and hospitality, but the Irish brand Barry's Tea is one of my very favorite black teas.

HOW MUCH?

How much tea does it take for an anti-cancer effect? That's the million dollar question. We all want to know just how much tea we need to drink to get our "I'll crush you, cancer!" posture on, and help reduce our risk of onset, progress or relapse of disease. In looking to tea for its therapeutic benefits, we need to take into account all of the most current quantitative scientific data available. Not all potential health problems can be averted, of course, but we all have a great deal more control over our wellness than we might be acting on. Tea is not the silver bullet panacea. It won't wipe out the effects of a pack-a-day smoking habit, hormone replacement therapy or any other risk patterns which have been indicated to increase the risk of disease, but drinking tea daily can help fuel your immune system to a better state of readiness for whatever curve balls might come your way.

The good news is that the research indicates you only need to consume 1 to 1.2 L (a little more than one quart) of freshly steeped whole leaf tea each day to bask in its therapeutic benefits. **That's a five-cup-a-day tea habit**, or in today's "bigger is better" society, just three mugs of tea. If you drink this much throughout the day, every day, your body could enjoy a significant increase in plasma antioxidant capacity, which can mean the beginning of a reduction in DNA damage in your cells. Some studies have shown those benefits being measurable in as little as one week of drinking 6 cups (1.4 L) of tea a day. Remember, your body is stunningly amazing, and it's just waiting to respond positively to every advantage you bring its way. And guess what? The higher per capita tea drinking nations consume on the average of four to six servings throughout the day. I find it interesting that those tea drinkers naturally nail the recommended amount right on the head. Keep in mind that too much of anything turns out to be not such a good thing, and that anything in excess won't be good for you. As positive as your five servings of tea are for maintaining wellness, doubling or tripling that amount isn't a good idea, and can start to become toxic to your cells.

Your total caffeine intake is also an important thing to keep tabs on. Each 8 ounce (240 ml) serving of white or green tea will give you between 10 mg and 35 mg of caffeine. Black tea will provide 40 mg to 50 mg of caffeine per 8 ounce (240 ml) serving. Pu-erh tea can get up as high as 60 mg of caffeine per serving, which is approximately half as much caffeine as a same-size cup of coffee. Note that some of those imposter ready-to-drink energy beverages are packing more than 200 mg of caffeine. The Academy of Nutrition and Dietetics says that 300 mg of caffeine per day won't have any negative effects on most people. Some negative side effects of having too much caffeine aren't fun, and can include anxiety, fast breathing, difficulty sleeping, headache, irregular heartbeat, nausea, vomiting and tremors.

HOW OFTEN?

Your body absorbs tea nutrients best when you drink them on an empty stomach. EGCg has a better chance of making it into your bloodstream without degradation when it doesn't come into contact with local bacteria in your gut. This makes tea a perfect pre-breakfast drink, but you may have some difficulty sucking down green tea on an empty stomach. Make sure you try teas from different regions, as they'll likely all work differently on your gut. If you're obsessed with drinking green teas and they just aren't working out for you, give yourself a break and start with a big mug of a favorite black tea in the morning. Remember, they're all good.

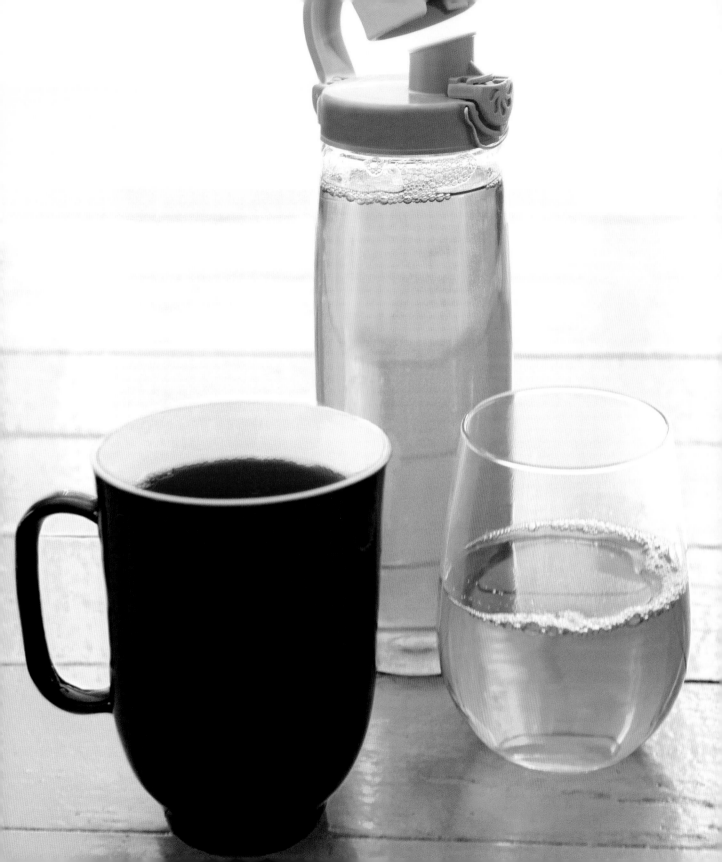

You want to keep a high tea polyphenol level in your bloodstream at all times. Studies show that timing is important in getting this right. When you drink tea, the peak concentrations of polyphenols in your cells happen one and two hours later. Those levels then come down gradually, and come down to essentially nil within 24 hours. **So sip your tea consistently throughout the day**—the benefits can be observed in improved blood vessel function in as quickly as a half hour after you drink it.

After six weeks of tea consumption, your body may show lower levels of the stress hormone cortisol and greater subjective relaxation, together with reduced platelet activation. Translation: Drinking tea helps you recover more rapidly from stress. This extends to when you drink tea immediately post-exercise, its rich antioxidant content can help boost recovery and limit oxidative stress to muscles. Observers of the athletic scene sometimes wonder if it's more than a coincidence that some of the best endurance athletes in the world—the Kenyan runners—sip tea throughout the day. And FYI, they always drink it hot.

So to get the full benefits bang from your tea, start with it early in the day and sip often, between meals and especially pre- and post-exercise.

HOW DRINKING HOT BEVERAGES CAN KEEP YOU COOL

Morocco and tea go hand in hand. Like with almost every strong tea-drinking culture, tea is considered a gesture of hospitality in Morocco and is almost always offered as a welcome to guests, traditionally prepared by the male head of the family. Just as in China, there's no such thing as getting through a business discussion or negotiation session in Marrakesh without taking some time to sit down for glass of delicious hot and sweet Moroccan mint Nana tea. The glasses are small (about 4 ounces [120 ml]), straight and cylindrical in design with elaborate ornamentation (think henna). You may have seen images of tea being poured by Moroccans using the ragwa method, from way up high. Many will tell you that's done to aerate the tea and create some delightful aroma and foam on top of the tea, but I've also heard that since it's the male head of household pouring the tea, that this gesture came from an intention to lift and flaunt the teapot higher than any neighbors' teapots. Bottom line—the teapots are indeed sexy and beautiful, and taking tea Moroccan-style can feel like restorative aromatherapy.

Moroccan-style green tea is served hot, with fresh mint leaves added. This makes it light and refreshing, even if you've just finished a hot day's trek through the mountains or desert. It's surprising, but hot beverages can actually cool you down. When your brain gets the message "TOO HOT" from sipping a warm beverage, it sets in motion the mechanisms to help cool you off, which causes you to begin to sweat. If you're not wearing massive layers of clothing, the sweat has somewhere to evaporate to, thus cooling you down. I always wondered why Russian ballet dancers would gather around their steaming thermos after rehearsals. Same goes for the Kenyan runners you see in my hometown of Boulder, Colorado, who are often sipping hot tea after a workout. Both cases made me wonder if they didn't trust the water without boiling it, but as turns out, they probably just knew more than I did about how to keep cool. Note: When you're sipping hot tea on a winter hike, it's actually warming you up. Your body is cold and doesn't get to the point where it sends that "TOO HOT" message to your brain.

You can find the recipe for Unsweetened Moroccan Mint on page 173 in Chapter 10.

IF YOU THINK WELLNESS IS EXPENSIVE, TRY CANCER

According to numbers released by the American Cancer Society (ACS), cancer's price tag is upwards of $895 billion, a sum that represents 1.5 percent of the world's gross domestic product (GDP). This is just its toll in terms of disability and productive years of life lost and doesn't even begin to take into account the cost of curing and managing the disease from a medical perspective. The ACS report claims that cancer's cost to society is more than that of human immunovirus (HIV), malaria, the flu and all other communicable diseases combined. Of course, further research is needed to continue to seek more effective ways of combating cancer, but so many straight-forward, and even cost-saving measures can be taken to set many potential patients on the road to prevention.

If we look at this issue from a global economic perspective, the impetus in favor of encouraging and enabling simple preventive measures seems clear. Just imagine if you could take one percent of the GDP lost to cancer in the U.S. and use that to replace less-healthy beverages in public high schools with fresh whole-leaf tea—it would save money in the end, right? But is it realistic to expect that a premium cup of tea can wean people off sweetened, carbonated, chemically enhanced and frozen creamy and fatty beverages? Does this translate to an equally smart investment on a personal level? Ultimately, we are responsible for our own wellness. What's it worth to you?

THE COST OF A DAILY TEA HABIT

Let's take a look at this from both ends of the spectrum: luxury-loving wellness lady and frugal health fanatic. Most of us will probably fall somewhere in between, so this will give us the upper and lower bounds by which to understand what a tea habit will cost.

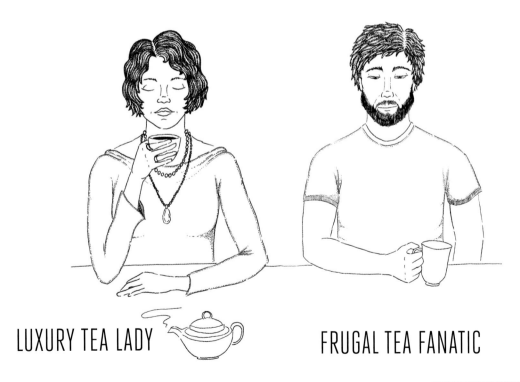

LUXURY TEA LADY   FRUGAL TEA FANATIC

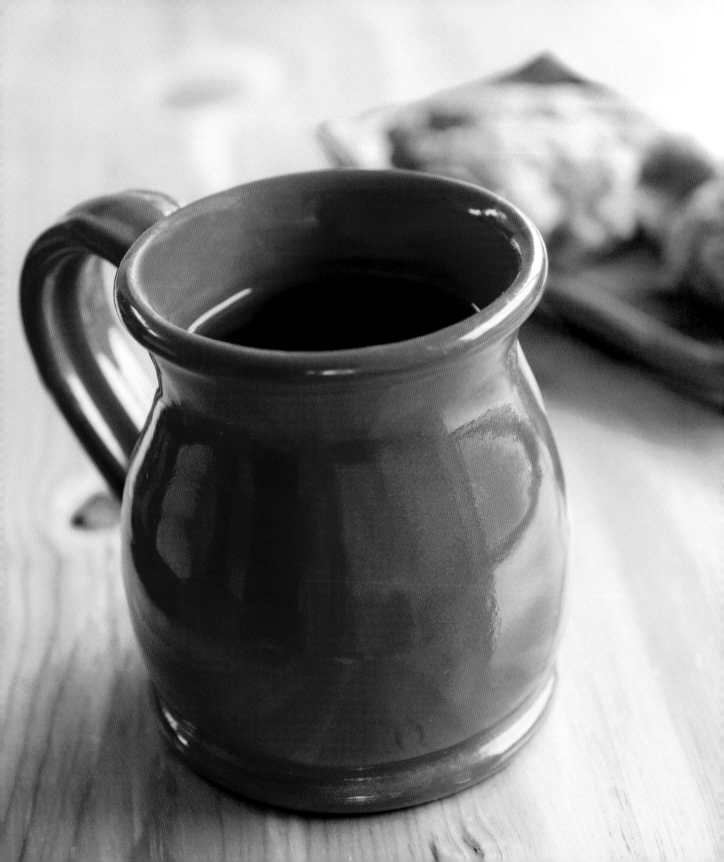

Luxury tea lady wants to treat herself to only the highest quality teas. After all, if she's going to become a regular tea drinker she may as well become a connoisseur. She might choose to start her mornings with a fine Japanese gyokuro green tea of fine deep emerald leaves grown at the base of Mount Fuji. Mid-morning, she's going to whip up a latte with ceremonial-grade matcha green tea (half an hour before her workout), giving her a boost and maximizing the burn from her gym time. With lunch, she'll enjoy some freshly brewed iced ginger peach black tea. Mid-afternoon, this lucky lady is going to break into an aged pu-erh tea from Yunnan, China, because she wants to work off whatever fat she can from her lunch, without needing to head back to the gym. And then there's tea time with her girlfriends. The hip come to sip at her place now, so she'd better treat them to something special, so let's make it a Taiwanese oolong.

Gyokuro green tea	$160/lb, or $0.70/serving
Ceremonial grade matcha	$20/oz, or $0.70/serving
Gourmet ginger peach tea	$35/lb, or $0.15/serving
Aged pu-erh tea	$57/lb, or $0.25/serving
Oolong tea	$115/lb, or $0.50/serving
Daily tea expense: $2.30	

Frugal tea fanatic just wants to get the job done. His preference would be to get an equivalent (or better) dose of tea polyphenols as the fancy lady, without all the fancy flavors, names and price tags. He's starting the day with a strong mug of gunpowder green tea. Next, he too will be downing some matcha green tea, maybe in a homemade energy drink. Let's make it a double dose—frugal's not really up for taking five tea timeouts a day if he can get it done in fewer steeps. Mid-afternoon, he'll have an iced sencha green tea to avoid the afternoon slump. He'll finish up with an Assam black tea in the late afternoon.

Gunpowder green tea	$23/lb, or $0.10/serving
Matcha green tea	$66/half-lb, or $0.60/2 servings
Sencha green tea	$34/lb, or $0.15/serving
Assam black tea	$23/lb, or $0.10/serving
Daily tea expense: $0.95	

Bottom line: You can get an amazingly diverse and healthful mix of five servings of tea daily for as little as $30 a month, and beyond that, you can splurge as little or as much as you'd like and your budget will allow. Even the most lavish tea habit, if you steep the tea yourself, amounts to less than the cost of a couple of shots of espresso or a coffee from your local coffee shop.

EASY WAYS TO SNEAK TEA INTO YOUR EVERY DAY

Begin your day with tea, as this is the best time of day for your body to absorb its benefits. Even if you need to grab a coffee an hour later, you're rousing your cells with tea polyphenols, which you can't get anywhere else.

Cold brew, and sip throughout the day. Get a large water bottle, and fill it with your favorite cold brew every morning. Choose a low-caffeine tea, and this becomes your new enriched water.

Keep calm, as the British say, and get an afternoon tea habit going.

SO WHAT'S THE BIG DEAL WITH AFTERNOON TEA ANYWAY?

Anna, the seventh Duchess of Bedford, was apparently a woman unwilling to accept the afternoon doldrums. As was the custom in 18th century England, Anna would have a huge breakfast, a meal hardly worth calling lunch and then wait until 8 o'clock or later before sitting down to a substantial dinner. Those of us who eat a snack at our desks and then rush off after work to pick up kids, the dry cleaning and groceries and then begin cooking dinner at 7 o'clock know exactly how she felt when she described the sinking feeling she got around 5 o'clock.

Today, many of us would reach for a smoothie or an energy bar. Being a Duchess, however, Anna chose to combat this lull in energy and spirit by sitting down to a nice cup of tea accompanied by sandwiches and cakes. The idea was such a good one that soon her friends and acquaintances began joining her, and afternoon tea became a ritual. Over time, the staff caught on as well, and eventually two very distinct versions came into being. High tea was embraced by the working class who served up whopping plates of food alongside a nice strong cuppa. It was a more substantial meal, essentially dinner. Low tea, quite contrary to its title, was the showy, ostentatious and rather less nutritious version of tea that was served to the aristocrats. Here the emphasis was more on the linens and china than on the beverage or accompanying foods. No doubt this low tea is where the stiff pinky finger first began poking out from the side of teacups. The names derive from the height of the tables on which the meals were served. High tea was served on higher (working) tables and low tea was on tables that we would call coffee tables.

Whether high or low, afternoon tea became as much a social phenomenon as it was a culinary trend. Today's re-emerging interest in afternoon tea is also a social movement, a revolt against the high-octane beverages and fast-paced living in which too many of us find ourselves enmeshed. For both our physical and spiritual well-being, an afternoon tea break is an inviting and joyful luxury. As Henry James said in his novel *Portrait of a Lady*, "There are few hours in my life more agreeable than the hour dedicated to the ceremony known as afternoon tea."

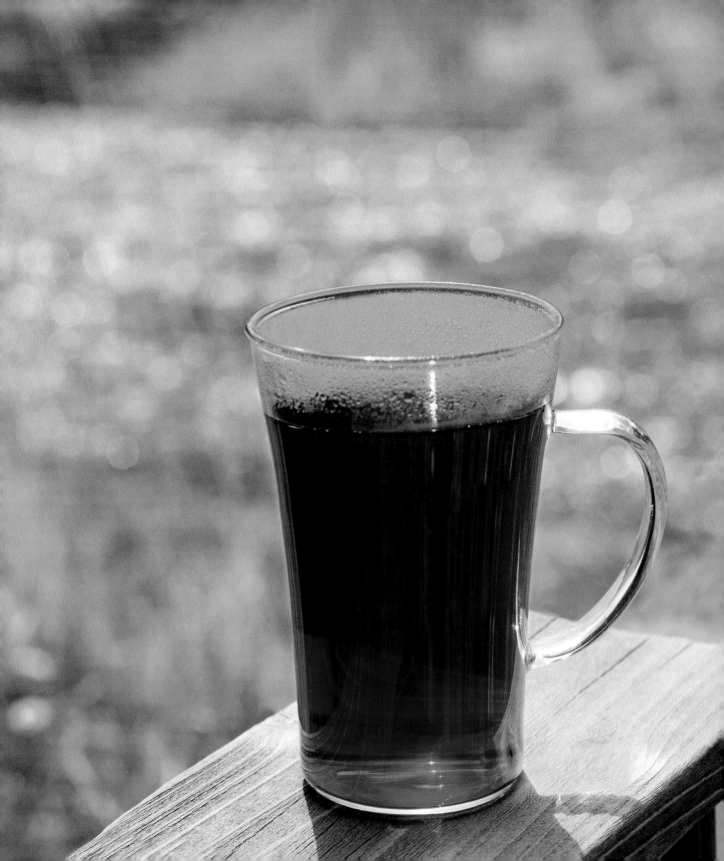

Chapter 4

GRAB YOUR HEALTH BY THE BOWLS

THE MORE YOU GET, THE MORE YOU WANT

Kathryn Kloberdanz's story

I received my breast cancer diagnosis the week of September 11, 2001. It didn't make sense that anyone should be overly concerned about me having cancer when so many thousands were killed in such horrible tragedies. At that same time, my dad's health was crashing. I had an overwhelming feeling of despair. I went through the motions of fighting the cancer, but I felt stunned by everything that was happening around me. Of course, I cried many tears, and it was traumatic to have both my boobs cut off in the coming months, but my dad's death during that same period hurt me more deeply than my personal struggles. I could get breast implants and try to look somewhat normal, but I couldn't bring him back to life.

Before breast cancer, I loved playing tennis, and my tennis girlfriends were my closest community. After surgery, the first thing I asked was, "When can I play tennis again?" The response was, "As soon as you want," but that didn't turn out to be the case. I couldn't hold my own purse, or drive, or do anything with my arms for months. After some hugely therapeutic rehab with a wonderfully caring yoga teacher, I can enjoy playing tennis now, but my game has never come back to the same level. Keeping a gentle yoga practice is a mainstay in my life to help me.

Six years after my recovery, I realized my life was all work and no play. On a whim, I tried drumming, which then led me to the marimba. The marimba music made my heart sing, but handling the larger mallets for some of the instruments required me to build strength and do special stretches that I'd learned from yoga. My passion for playing led me to re-organize my work life so that I could spend more time doing things I love.

Breast cancer was a huge gift to me. It was the kick in the butt that made me learn how to stand up for myself. I learned in time to become my own defiant self-advocate, and I learned how to make my own choices for dealing with my body. That attitude has stayed with me post-disease. I know how to take steps to accept what is, how to remember to honor my values and to pursue what makes me happy. Yes, my body image has experienced a great assault—and yet my life is richer than ever—and, get this: I'm in a marimba band now, for Pete's sake!

THE ANTIOXIDANT POWERHOUSE

If you were offered something that worked like a green tea army on steroids, would you drink it? Hell yeah, you're thinking . . . Carpe that Diem! The obvious way to take full advantage of green tea's potential would be to eat the whole leaf. But you're probably not ready to start munching on tea leaves like a panda bear working on bamboo, right? Fortunately, there's a much more elegant solution.

Matcha (pronounced MAH-cha) is pure green tea powder. It's just straight stone-ground tea leaves. When you drink matcha, you're not just drinking the water-soluble molecules that steep their way out of the leaf into your cup. It's a diffusion, as opposed to an infusion of green tea leaves, so **you're actually ingesting the whole tea leaf**. Now put that in your bowl and sip on it. Yep, matcha is traditionally prepared and served in a bowl. And by traditionally, I mean for the past 1,000 plus years. The Chinese were the first to dry and pulverize green tea into a fine powder. They called it Tea Mud, and prepared it by whisking the powdered tea in a bowl with water. Eventually, this practice was abandoned in China, but not before traveling Zen monks from Japan picked it up. The tea seeds they brought back and started growing in Japan were cared for with entirely new and different traditions of cultivation and processing, and with time, Japan blossomed into one of the top tea cultures in history. Powdered green matcha tea has been an immutable part of Japanese culture since the 13th century, and today it's still one of the nation's most prized beverages.

Zen monks probably didn't spend much of their time worrying about cancer, but they did know about how to live long, stress-free lives. One of their secrets was drinking matcha green tea, which helped them stay alert, yet calm, during long hours of meditation. Their practice evolved into the classic Japanese tea ceremony called *Cha-do*, which translates as "Tea-way." The Way of Tea, as we refer to it, is a ceremonial preparation and presentation of matcha, established by the great 16th century tea master, Sen no Rikyu, in a blend of Zen and Taoist principles. It's a beautiful tradition in which the tea powder is solemnly whisked into a frothy, sweet and umami beverage in a specific preparation and serving bowl. Japanese tea ceremony is a harmonious and tranquil experience of appreciation, done while both host and guest maintain a spirit of mutual grace, beauty and etiquette. There's a quote from Okakura Kakuzo, an early 20th century tea master, which I think embodies the spirit of the ceremony, "Perfection is everywhere if we only choose to recognize it."

The history of this tea ceremony even has a macabre story. During the Second World War, Japanese kamikaze pilots would participate in a tea ceremony when they were called to fly their suicide mission. That perfect bowl of frothed green tea would be their final drink. A 15th-generation Japanese grand tea master named Soshitsu Sen was one of the pilots in the kamikaze squadron and performed these tea ceremonies. Interestingly enough, the war ended before his number was picked.

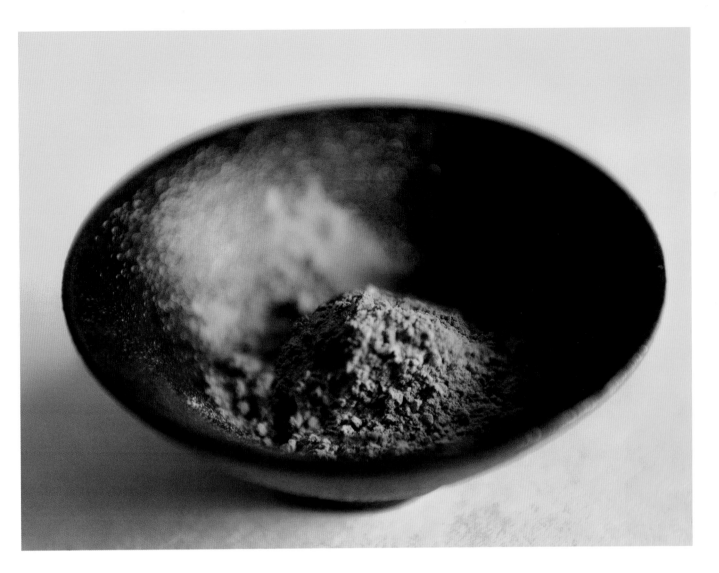

WHY MATCHA?

So why are we so concerned with the Japanese tea ceremony? It's because a single serving of matcha can give you several times the antioxidants of a cup of infused whole leaf tea. This is the shortcut I mentioned earlier: If you were in a real time bind to chase down your daily tea polyphenols, you could just slurp down five servings-worth in a couple of bottles of cold brew matcha that took you 10 seconds to shake up. Now that's convenient! It's like getting in the green tea catechin fast lane. Gram for gram, matcha has about twice the total EGCg content of whole leaf green tea. Matcha gives you more than 30 times the vitamin C you get in whole leaf green tea. The protein and calcium values of matcha dwarf that of infused green tea—they're about 200 times higher, and the iron content is more than 50 times higher. Yup, **matcha's just like drinking your vegetables**.

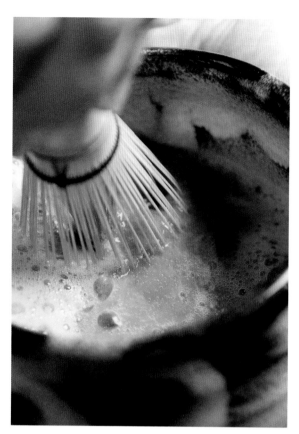

THE TECHNICAL STUFF

The granddaddy of Japanese tea cultivation, Zen priest Esai, wrote a two-volume book in 1211 titled *How to Stay Healthy by Drinking Tea*. It opens with the sentence: "Tea is the ultimate mental and medical remedy and has the ability to make one's life more full and complete." So even if 13th century Zen monks didn't spend much of their time thinking about cancer, they still knew a heck of a lot more than most of us about what tea can do for your health. Which approach would you expect gets you more antioxidants from tea: steeping the leaves in boiling or near-boiling water, then discarding the leaves and drinking the resulting infusion, or just eating pure ground tea leaves?

Matcha is made from very fine tea grown under the most controlled conditions. No surprises here—the star of the Japanese tea ceremony isn't going to be found growing wild on some hillside. Japanese tea leaves destined to be made into matcha spend part of their growing cycle in the shade. At the appropriate time for harvesting, the shaded tea leaves are hand-picked. Once the leaves are picked, they're steamed until completely dried, which contributes to matcha's almost electric green color. Matcha leaves are never rolled or kneaded—their stems are removed, leaving only the finest part of the leaves. The final step of grinding the leaves into a fine green powder is done using a granite wheel (think giant mortar and pestle). Cutting down on sunlight maximizes the amount of chlorophyll in the leaves, and chlorophyll-rich leaves tend to be darker green in color. They taste more grassy than Chinese green teas, which are generally cultivated in higher sunlight conditions. The shade is also what gives Japanese green teas their pleasant savory, vegetal, edging toward seaweed-like flavor. There's even a term for it: Umami. Umami is described as one of the five basic tastes, along with sweetness, sourness, bitterness and saltiness. It's an unmistakable taste sensation, which can be described as long-lasting, mouthwatering and slightly astringent on the tongue.

HOW TO MAKE A PERFECT BOWL OF MATCHA

Pure matcha tea powder and authentic, traditional tea ceremony tools are the easiest way to set yourself up to develop the skills you'll need to whip up a fresh and inviting bowl of matcha. You can find these in most Asian stores, tea boutiques or online. Matcha comes in many grades and prices. The first time I bought a low-grade (but well-priced) matcha and whisked it up with a fork in water that was probably too hot, I damn near passed the tea through my nose when I tried it. With better quality matcha and a little practice, you can perfect your technique and turn out a sweet and frothy bowl of this antioxidant-rich gourmet tea for yourself or your guests. Master the matcha act, and you'll be in the company of just a handful of tea sommeliers in this country.

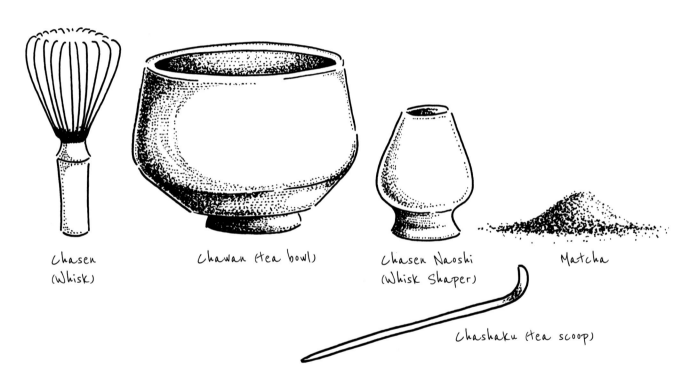

Chasen (Whisk)

Chawan (tea bowl)

Chasen Naoshi (Whisk Shaper)

Matcha

Chashaku (tea scoop)

The essential tools for making an authentic bowl of matcha are: tea bowl (chawan), tea scoop (chashaku) and tea whisk (chasen).

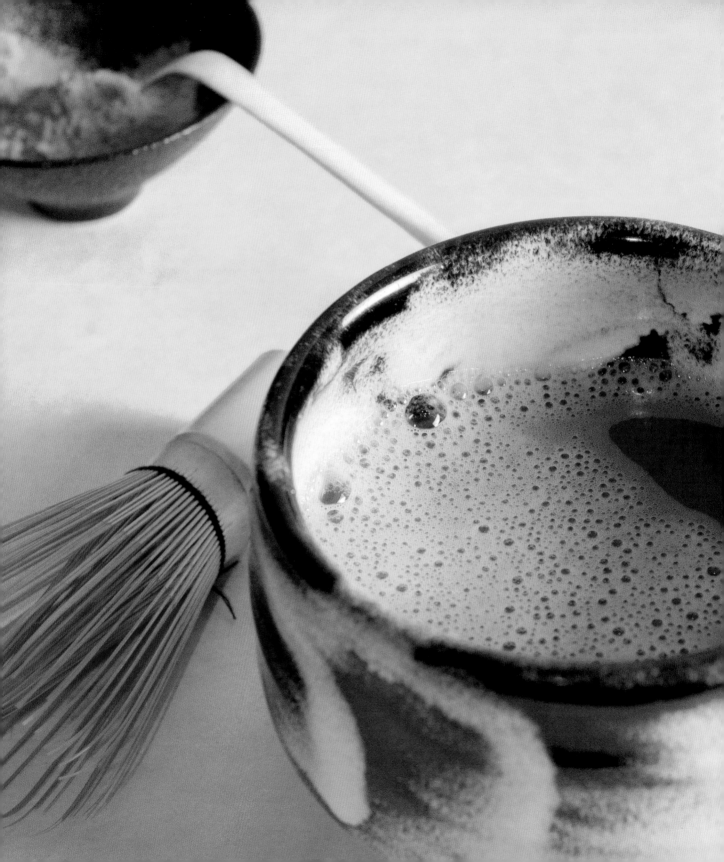

The traditional bamboo tea whisk helps dissolve the green tea powder completely into the water, frothing the beverage to make a consistent, well blended and aromatic bowl of matcha. Once you've successfully whisked your first great bowl of traditional ceremonial matcha in your own kitchen, you'll be truly smitten by this green elixir which embodies harmony, respect, purity and tranquility. An amazing bonus given that we started down the matcha route for wellness and longevity.

A key point is to not skimp on the quality of your matcha green tea powder. This is not for the sake of tea snobbery. Matcha is expensive to begin with. It's also the tea that requires the most precise proportions, water temp and water quality to turn out a tasty product. Spending the extra pennies per serving on this one could make or break your chances of falling for a seriously healthy habit. You'll be using about half as much by weight per serving, compared with leaf tea. A rounded teaspoon of green tea leaves weighs approximately two grams, and a single serving of matcha is one half teaspoon, which weighs about one gram.

SOME TIPS FOR TURNING OUT GOOD MATCHA

Make sure the color is more green (looks fresh) than army-khaki (been stored too long).

Don't buy a matcha that looks clumpy. And if you did, sift it. Seriously, you'll thank yourself when whisking.

If possible, buy organic. After all, you are actually eating it.

Make sure your matcha comes from Japan. After 1,000 years, they've got this down, like no one else. If it doesn't say Japan, you can assume it's not from there, because putting that on the label allows it to be sold at a premium.

Keeping your matcha tea powder fresh is key, so store it in an air-tight container in a cool place, keep it away from any moisture and direct light, and keep it away from any items with a strong odor.

Proportions are critical—rounded ½ teaspoon (1 g) and ½ cup (120 ml) of fresh water.

Use a two step process for mixing—make a paste first, then add the rest of the water.

The water temperature should be approximately 160 to 170°F (70 to 75°C).

Froth with a loose wrist whisking motion.

MAKING THE PERFECT MATCHA

1. Measure out ½ cup (120 ml) boiling water into a measuring cup and allow it to cool for 3 to 4 minutes, until it's barely too hot to the touch (that should be about 160–170°F [70–75°C]). This is key! Matcha made with water that's too hot is not only bitter, but will provide less vitamin C. While you're waiting for the water to cool, preheat your matcha bowl by filling it half full with hot water. Discard that water before going to Step 2.

2. Place ½ teaspoon (1 g) of matcha powder into your the bowl and add 1 tablespoon (15 ml) of the water from your measuring cup to it. Mix the powder into the water vigorously with your whisk, until you have a smooth, pasty mixture.

3. Add the rest of the hot water from the measuring cup, and whisk the matcha into a nice frothy drink by flicking your wrist in a back and forth zigzag motion. Whisk through the center point of the bowl with each pass. Your grip on the whisk should stay light, to keep your wrist free and relaxed. Keep turning the bowl slowly with your non-whisking hand, or alternate the direction of your whisking motion, to mix and oxygenate all the liquid in the bowl. This usually takes about 100 back-and-forth whisking moves. Hang in there—you got this! (P.S.: You can also froth your matcha with a milk foamer, available for under $5.) Now drink up while it's nicely frothed.

Give yourself a chance to get used to matcha's flavor. It may take a few tries before you've trained your taste buds to crave it straight. Matcha is naturally sweeter than steeped leaf green teas, and although the taste will hit most of us Westerners as something totally peculiar the first time around, most people will admit that it's actually strangely appealing.

THICK VERSUS THIN MATCHA

Once you get into drinking matcha, your mood and your palate will guide you as to how much water you want to add. Thick matcha (koicha) is what the stronger version with less water is called, and thin matcha (usucha) is the less intense one. You may find yourself wanting different strengths of matcha, depending on the time of day, your energy level or your mood. I can't drink strong matcha first thing in the morning on an empty stomach, but I do like to start my day with matcha, so I make it pretty thin. If I'm drinking it in the afternoon, I prefer it stronger. Go with your gut! Even though it's antioxidant-rich and good for you, matcha can be enjoyed for the excellent gourmet tea that it is, and not as though you're drinking medicine. But, if you feel you need a "spoonful of sugar" to make it go down, a good gateway drink to a fresh-frothed bowl of matcha is a matcha latte or smoothie, which introduces the intense power of this emerald mixture to your palate gradually.

MY JAPANESE TEA CEREMONY "AHA" MOMENT

When visiting Tokyo, you can't help but feel smacked right between the eyes by leading-edge technology, fashion and consumerism. But even amidst the crazy pace and pop culture that sometimes feels more like a pressure cooker than a zen garden, traditional culture is highly respected and practiced. Kabuki theater performances are in full swing, traditional architecture that survived World War II is carefully maintained and revered, and one of the hottest museums is Tokyo-Edo, a beautiful modern complex in the Sumo-wrestler stables neighborhood, which showcases old Tokyo.

One of my trips to Japan coincided with an annual event, the Tokyo Grand Tea Ceremony. This very grand tea ceremony is a tradition that you might think would be losing attention to Italian espresso and Parisian-style tea in this city. But it's actually alive and well, and practiced by many dedicated young apprentices studying with the older tea mistresses of Tokyo. The three main schools of tea ceremony in Japan all share Sen no Rikyu, the originator of The Way of Tea, as their founder. The number of people practicing tea ceremony at home has declined dramatically over the past few decades as Japanese homes and patterns became more Westernized. Many people even lost the skill of sitting kneeling down, which is how all tea ceremony has been traditionally taught. In recent years, however, there's been a resurgence of interest in the traditional tea ceremony in schools, both public and private.

I was so excited to get to go to this big public tea ceremony that I was the first visitor to arrive. Those who know me well would undoubtedly think I had my watch stuck in the wrong time zone . . . but my enthusiasm clearly flattered my hosts, and I was given the first seat in the front row. I'd be lying if I said I was basking in my front and center observer-guest location. The ceremony was scheduled to last an hour, and I wasn't sure how my attention span would hold up. Seriously, you couldn't help but wonder what could possibly be going on for an hour to prepare and serve a bowl of tea. What was up with all the formality? Why so many tools to complicate this process? And finally, why in the world is this being done and spectated upon by so many people?!

The setting for this event was in the teahouse of my favorite park in Tokyo, called Hamarikyu. It's a tidal garden on the Sumigawa river, the site of a former Shogun's duck-hunting property. Every view you can take in this garden is picture-perfect. Japanese landscape architecture has always struck me as a collection of perfectly balanced scenes. It's impossible to take a bad photo here, because no matter where you point your camera, the composition is perfect. This concept of perfect balance carried over to the tea ceremony, where first the host, then each participant, comes on the scene in perfect timing and pitch. Even in the stillness, there was a sense of movement. Beauty, respect, humility and appreciation were communicated with graceful gestures. This harmony was further carried through to the balance of flavors between the smooth, but bitter, whipped matcha and the ultra-delicate seasonal sweets offered before and with the tea. It's customary for these melt-in-your-mouth treats to be made from local and seasonal fruits and shapes (ours were shaped like maple leaves and had fall-harvest plum flavors sandwiched in delicate wafers). Each one in isolation would be delicious, but the tea and sweets together were purely perfect. And guess what? This beautifully-paced choreographed event was over in what felt like just a brief instant. Perhaps this was one of my first forays into meditation, seeing the beauty in the mundane and feeling complete tranquility during my busy travels within this busiest of cities. In any case, it's a treasured memory I won't ever forget.

YES, MATCHA IS A SUPERFOOD

We know that matcha is packed with green tea cancer-bashing catechins. Let's take a look at all the other things that make matcha a superfood.

For starters, you ingest and eat matcha. Since tea is a plant-based beverage, you can think of it as taking straight phytochemicals. It is, in fact, a food. It has protein and fiber, and two rounded teaspoons (4 g) of matcha contain a gram of protein. You can't just tell your protein powder to move and get out the way, but matcha does add a protein boost to your smoothies and rapidly absorbable dietary fiber in every serving. Soluble fiber improves digestive health and can help to keep blood sugar levels in check. Yep, this mean green powder is good for keeping things regular, and supermodels have blatantly vouched for it.

Each serving of matcha yields about 30 times as much vitamin C as a steeped leaf green tea. That's a great combo with the other natural antioxidants in green tea, if you're ever feeling cold symptoms or weakness coming on. Per teaspoon (2 g), you get the same amount of natural vitamin C from matcha as you do from fresh lemon juice.

Remember the part about the tea that's ground into matcha spending time in the shade? That not only boosts the concentration of chlorophyll but the tea-exclusive amino acid theanine in those leaves as well. Matcha has four times the theanine of steeped green tea per serving. That can also help to explain why the caffeine effects of matcha may not feel as intense as other green teas.

Not only does chlorophyll make matcha so bright and pretty, it's really good for you (think liquid sunshine). It's a powerful detoxifier with anti-bacterial properties and its own arsenal of antioxidants. Chlorophyll is highly alkaline, and its high oxygen content helps deliver more oxygen to the blood. It's used in traditional medicine to help clear the body of toxins and balance blood pH levels, and it is the main reason people pay $5 or more for shots of wheatgrass. But matcha's much nicer and classier to drink, so go grab a bowl and get whisking.

For all that matcha is, be leery of matcha antioxidant claims that sound unbelievable because they probably are! As wonderful and valid a product as matcha is, some of the numbers surrounding its antioxidant power are downright ridiculous. Merchants and magazines have tweeted and touted the claim that matcha has more than 100 times EGCg than regular green tea. This is simply not true and is a gross misrepresentation of what was actually in the referenced research: The EGCg content of matcha was over 100 times that of a low-end tea bag product, whose EGCg content was just plain piddly.

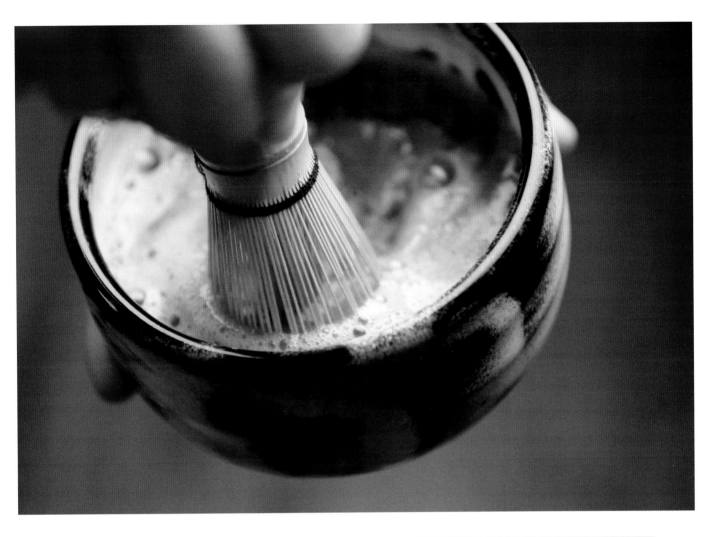

3 WAYS TO GET A QUICK HIT OF GREEN TEA CATECHINS

Getting one of your daily servings of tea with half a teaspoon of matcha in a bottle of water or a latte takes no time or effort at all. Matcha cold brews instantly. When you're feeling lazy about your tea prep, this is a fast and easy way to get it done!

- Shake a ½ teaspoon matcha up in your water bottle. Optional: Add a squeeze of lemon or lime.
- Shake a ½ teaspoon matcha up in a bottle of coconut water.
- Add a ½ teaspoon to a cold glass of milk, either cow or dairy-free.

PART THREE

MORE GREAT WAYS TO GIVE CANCER THE FINGER

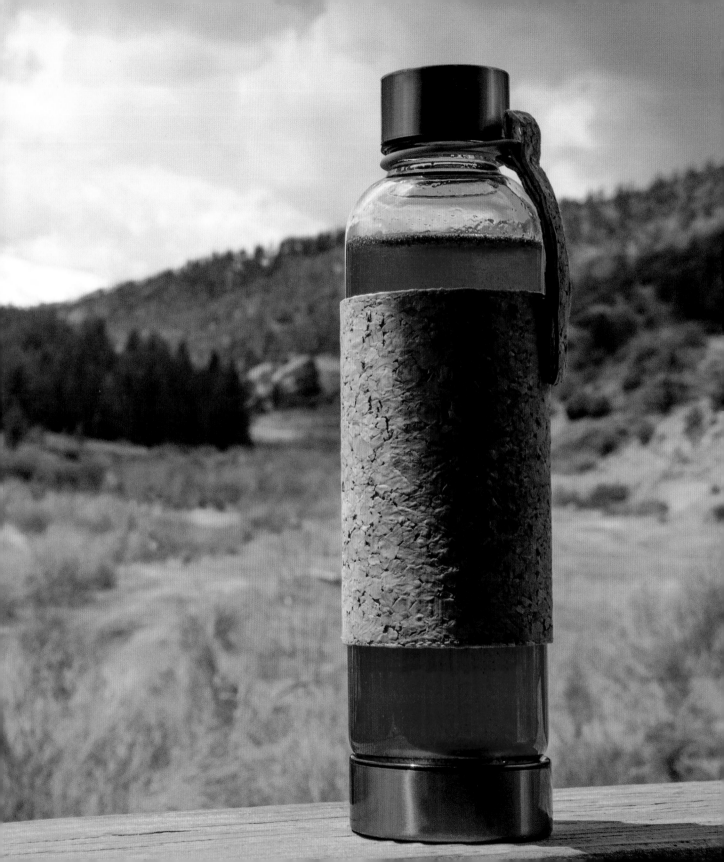

Chapter 5

CANCER HATES A HEALTHY HEART

FOLLOW YOUR HEART

Colorado Heartcycle

Colorado Heartcycle originally started in the 1970s with a group of cardiologists who were interested in what effects aggressive cycling at high altitude had on heart health. (Their findings were that it was not detrimental.) Over time, the group morphed into a nonprofit bicycling club that now offers supported tours around the country and even all over the world. Colorado Heartcycle guides over a dozen bike excursions each year, ranging from Fireworks of Fall on the Upper Hudson River to a Heart of Holland Bike & Barge tour and even a Mother, Daughter, Sister Tour with Love, Sweat & Gears, in the beautiful canyons and hot springs of Colorado.

Dr. Eugenia Miller, a cardiologist from Durango, Colorado, and a member of Heartcycle, offered her insights on the health benefits of exercise: "We know from lots of research over many years now that moderate regular exercise is very beneficial for heart health, hypertension and diabetes, both in terms of prevention and with respect to ameliorating pre-existing conditions. The American College of Sports Medicine and the American College of Cardiology have recognized that 30 minutes of moderate exercise daily, or more aggressive exercise for 75 minutes per week, is good for your health. It improves blood sugar and lipid levels, and has been found to reduce depression. Different exercise routines work best for different people. Some like to go to the gym, where they enjoy the social aspect and are inspired and encouraged by other people. There's a benefit to working out with others—it can make it more enjoyable, and is especially helpful with maintaining consistency in your commitment to exercise."

THE U.S. IS BROKENHEARTED

Heart disease outranks cancer as the number one killer of adults in the U.S. But you may be asking yourself, "What does cancer have to do with heart disease?" Hearts and tumors have a lot more in common than you might have ever guessed, and **keeping your heart healthy can actually lower your risk of cancer**. Cancer just hates that.

In a large-scale study of more than 6,000 men conducted at Duke University Medical Center, researchers found that those with heart disease had a 35 percent higher risk of prostate cancer. What's more, the risk became higher over time. By four years into the study, this same group of men's prostate cancer risk was 74 percent higher than for those with no evidence of coronary disease. Prostate cancer is the second-most deadly cancer for U.S. men behind lung cancer.

Another large scale study from the Northwestern University School of Medicine in Chicago determined that people who follow the American Heart Association's (AHA) seven heart health guidelines have a 51 percent lower risk of developing cancer than people who don't live by those guidelines. The study followed more than 13,000 healthy people's habits over 13 years. The Simple 7 heart health metrics were tracked and participants were screened for any cancer that developed during that time. What they found was that the more of these seven habits people followed, the less likely they were to develop cancer. Follow one habit and cancer risk was down by 20 percent. Follow five habits and bring cancer risk down by 38 percent. People who followed six of the seven heart health guidelines had a 51 percent lower cancer risk than the participants who didn't meet any of the steps. **This research informs us that you can control your health.**

Twenty years after the study began in 1987, researchers pulled hospital records and cancer registries and found that almost 22 percent of the participants had been diagnosed with lung, breast, prostate, colon or rectal cancer. And yes, those who had been diagnosed with cancer tended to follow fewer of the AHA's Simple 7 behaviors than those who didn't get the cancer diagnoses. Sure, we know that making smart lifestyle and diet choices are good for feeling better and living longer, but knowing that there's a connection between heart and cancer risk factors is downright awesome. Making a few simple adjustments can go a long way. Get motivated, but don't drive yourself crazy. Do a self-assessment (online at www.heart.org) and see which of the positive habits you already have down. For the habits you don't, take steps to tackle them one at a time. Keeping your disdain for cancer going strong can help you get motivated to make some amazing changes!

The concept which I've adopted that makes me feel like I can keep a healthy routine going is the 80/20 rule, which allows me to not beat myself up for eating or drinking bad things from time to time. It's totally changed my relationship with food. No more feelings of failure or despair, which are just plain toxic. The 80/20 lifestyle lets you take a break from being good 20 percent of the time. I just focus on the 80 percent, and the 20 percent takes care of itself. It's for those times when you're either traveling and eating out, or sharing food with friends or you just plain want an amazing dessert that might not be at the top of your healthy indulgences list. That's cool, as long as you allow yourself those splurges to happen only 20 percent of the time. For me, this works to help make healthy totally doable.

SHOW YOUR HEART YOU CARE

Here are the seven ways you can show your heart you care. And just so you know . . . a healthy heart loves to flip cancer the bird.

1. Just get off your butt.

Do 30 minutes of moderate physical activity at least five times a week. Or just be nice and take the dog for a walk when you get home from work. Sip on some tea 30 minutes before you head off to boost your burn.

2. Blast your belly.

About two-thirds of adults in the U.S. are overweight or obese. Excess fat, especially around the mid-section, is a health risk, so work on getting to and keeping a healthy weight. Hate crunches? Do some squats and planks. Re-hydrate with tea.

3. Eat smart.

A diet high in whole-grain fiber, lean proteins, colorful fruits and vegetables (and teas!) and low in saturated and trans fats, cholesterol, sodium and added sugars can greatly improve your health.

4. Ditch the soda pop and the sweet latte.

Keep safe blood sugar levels. Steep some tea instead and drink it straight.

5. Manage your cholesterol.

When you have too much low-density lipoprotein (LDL) cholesterol, plaque can form in your arteries and veins. This is bad news for your heart. Make sure you know where you stand. Green tea can help.

6. Chill out.

Keep blood pressure down. High blood pressure is the most significant risk for heart disease. Hibiscus herbal tea can help.

7. Don't smoke.

Period. Do whatever it takes. Make tea your habit.

Heart disease is mean. It claims one in every four adult deaths in the U.S. today. Cancer prevention aside, that fact alone makes it a very good idea to love and nurture your own heart to the max.

TEA IN PARIS ("TEEE IN PAREEE")

When you order tea in Paris, people assume that you're either trying to prove something (snob factor), or else that you have a medical problem (can't drink café). In my opinion, the French are quick to jump to assumptions, so you should view this reaction with some amusement. There are some pretty spectacular tea establishments in Paris that are snazzier than those romantic, cliché sidewalk cafés on every block. Anything the French set out to make chic, they make very, very chic. Just naturally. It's their damn way. Tea and over-the-top pastries are pretty devilishly fantastic in the city of lights, where culinary endeavors are taken most seriously. It shows in the tea. It's hard to get trash tea in Paris. This may be the only place in the world outside Asia where that's the case. It's ironic, in fact, that just across the English Channel the per capita consumption is so much higher, but the average quality is often mediocre. The French have made their tea their own. It's a little like a perfume shop, but it's quality teas. These will cater to your inner tea aficionado. If you're not OK with scented teas, you can still find your way to some great stuff. But I love to indulge in what the hottest local tea trends are. And guess what? You can just go on and pretend that pastry can't touch you when you're eating it in Paris. This country has the lowest incidence of heart disease in the world. P.S. Don't forget the red wine and dark chocolate with dinner, while you watch the Eiffel Tower twinkling . . .

TEA FOR A HEALTHY HEART

One of the many badass tea benefits uncovered by modern medical research is that high tea consumption leads to a healthier heart. I repeat: The very same teas you're drinking to tell cancer off make for a healthy heart.

The Seven Countries Study compared diet and lifestyle between seven contrasting countries and cultures for over half a century. The evidence showed that cardiovascular disease was preventable. After decades of follow-up, the study found that populations with higher than average flavonoid intake showed lower rates of heart disease. Elderly men who drank more than 4 cups (960 ml) of tea per day had a 60 percent lower risk of fatal coronary heart disease than those who drank less than 2 cups (480 ml) of per day. Middle-aged men who drank on average at least 5 cups (1.2 L) of tea per day had a 3 times lower stroke incidence than those who drank less than 2.5 cups (600 ml) per day. Now that'll get you drinking! Side note: The Seven Countries Study wasn't being sexist just for kicks—when they began their research in the 1950s, few women were dying of heart disease.

For some people, simply limiting cholesterol intake doesn't always significantly lower their blood cholesterol level. Green tea has been shown to help decrease cholesterol levels. In addition, research has shown that the free radical busting antioxidants in green tea may help prevent atherosclerosis, and in particular coronary artery disease. Researchers found that green tea can rapidly improve blood vessel function. Subjects experienced significant widening of their arteries in just 30 minutes after drinking the tea. Start steeping early in the day and sip often. You want to maintain the level of antioxidants in your bloodstream. Timing is everything.

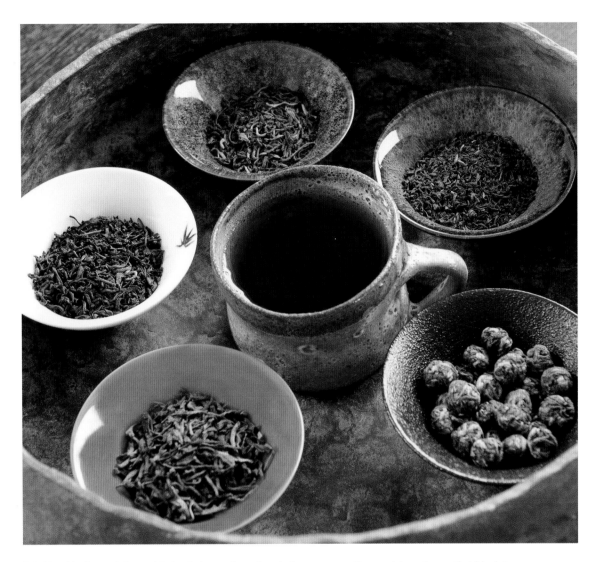

Drinking black tea daily could also help you keep heart disease away. Research has shown that black tea can improve vascular function in healthy individuals. Those improved effects are noticeable with just 1 cup (240 ml) per day and further improve by increasing the number of cups of tea consumed daily (the study tested up to 4 cups [960 ml] of black tea/day). The mix of polyphenol antioxidants and other compounds in black tea have their own unique heart-health benefits. One thing to keep in mind with black tea is that it has about two to three times the caffeine content of green tea. At about 40 to 60 mg of caffeine per serving, 5 cups (1.2 L) of black tea starts to add up. Remember that 300 mg/day is the caffeine threshold you want to watch out for. The side effects of consuming too much caffeine could actually end up doing your heart more harm than good.

ABOUT BLACK TEAS

Black tea is what most of the world (outside of China and Japan) drinks. It's what's in the fancy teacups of English royalty and Downton Abbey folk, as well as what you get in a glass of Southern sweet tea. One of the most recognizable teas to North American consumers is the spicy chai blend, prepared with milk. There are hundreds of varieties of black teas grown in more than 30 countries around the world. All tea types are available in a range of qualities from dusty machine-made bits to hand-picked whole leaf grade. Most black teas are harvested several times throughout the year. The Chinese refer to our black tea as red tea (Hong Cha) for the burgundy-red color of the infusion.

Green tea is the preferred tea in China while most black teas produced in China are geared for export. It's the Western world that actually got this tea on the map. In the early days of tea trade via caravan and ocean transport from China to Europe, green teas lost much of their quality of flavor and appearance along the way. So Chinese tea growers intentionally withered the tea leaves during processing, so they would be less likely to fade during the voyage west. The picked leaves were first let to wither naturally, before they were hand-twisted, rolled and broken, then exposed to air some more and finally completely dried out in heated woks. The end product was a darker twist on the classic Chinese green teas. Allowing the tea leaves to oxidize and turn black made freshness less of a factor and gave it a longer shelf life.

Chinese black tea leaves have been flavored since around the time the Ming Dynasty was founded in 1368, and have become wildly popular in America and Europe in recent decades. The addition of natural essences and flavors creates an exciting sensual and gastronomic experience, as both the tea and the scent are often enhanced in the mingling of the two. Tea can be flavored by adding fruits, floral essences and flavorings to the finished tea leaves. All tea leaves are very absorbent of fragrances. Popular scented black teas include Earl Grey, which is blended with bergamot; lapsang souchong, which is fragranced with pine wood smoke; rose tea, caramel tea and various fruit-flavored black teas.

India is the second largest tea exporter in the world. Like China, most of its tea production is consumed domestically. Although the same varietal of tea plant that makes the bold black teas in Southwestern China is indigenous to Northwestern India, tea was not a big part of the Indian diet until the British began producing tea there in the mid 19th century. The Indian palate was not satisfied by the British thin, sugared beverage, however. But by drawing from their own cultural pantry they created the tea drink that we know as chai. Every housewife and chaiwallah has his or her own recipe for what they call masala chai, or spice tea. Traditional Indian chai is a spicy, strong fragrant tea made on a strong black tea base simmered with ginger root, cardamom, cinnamon, allspice, peppercorns and cloves.

AND NOW FOR THE RINGERS!

Hibiscus

As a naturally caffeine-free herbal, hibiscus is a great way to stay healthfully hydrated any time of day. It offers a natural source of vitamin C and its own heap of antioxidants to give your immune system a boost, and it may be a heart-healthy dietary addition. Medical research shows that it's promising in treating high blood pressure and possibly, high cholesterol. Researchers found that six weeks of drinking hibiscus herbal tea each day could lower blood pressure in mildly hypertensive adults.

Hibiscus is the most common ingredient in herbal tea blends sold in the U.S. Grown throughout the tropics and subtropics of the world, hibiscus is a cooling and soothing floral which turns into a vibrant red infusion when brewed. Hibiscus tea tastes great cold-brewed. Mouthwatering, smooth and refreshing, it is ready to drink in less than ten minutes. Brewed hot, the taste of hibiscus flower petals is tart and exotic and reminiscent of fresh cranberries. This is a beautiful and refreshing herbal, and is a great choice for healthy hydration year-round.

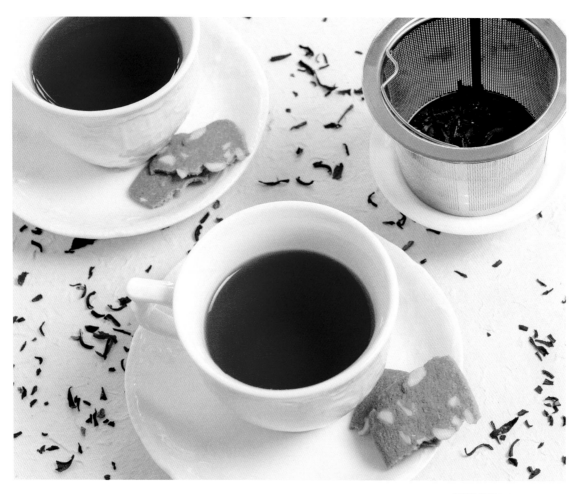

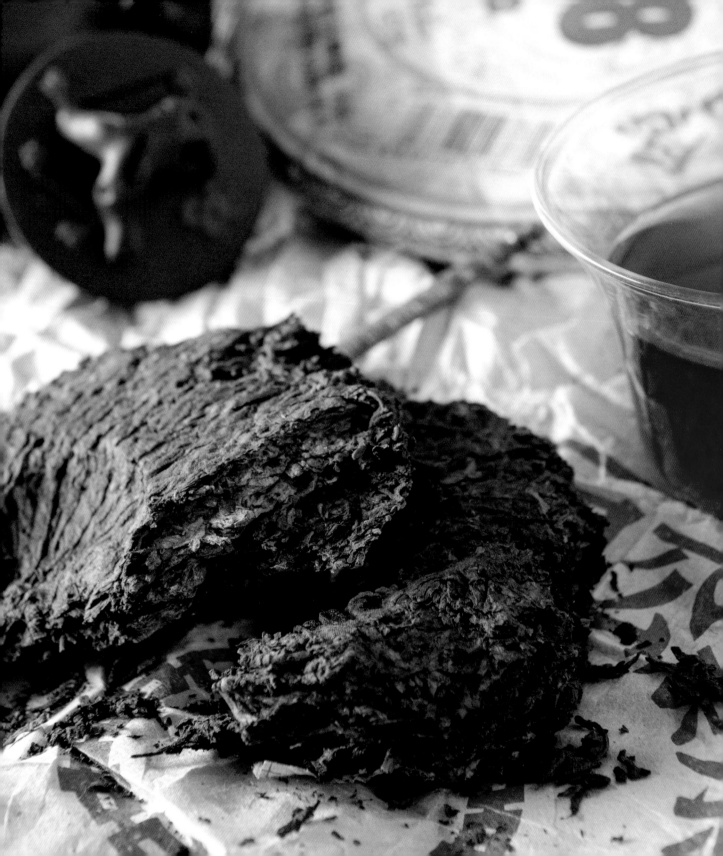

MY PU-ERH LOVE AFFAIR

My affair with pu-erh began with my very first sip at the Rocky Mountain Tea Festival here in Boulder, Colorado, about 15 years ago. It was love at first sip! To me, this was the most luxurious hot beverage I'd ever tasted: earthy, bold, robust and smooth, like curling up under an exotic and comfortable blanket. But most of the other seminar participants, including my then-teenage girls, were not in agreement. One of my daughters spat it out into Boulder Creek and said, "I could find everything you need to make this tea right in my own backyard compost pile." It was surprising to me that not everyone was falling for these infusions at the corner of drinkable and thinkable, made from tea cakes with names such as Camel's Breath.

What makes pu-erh so peculiar and unique is that it's processed in such a way that the oxidation doesn't completely stop after the leaves are dried. With this continued microbial fermentation going on, pu-erh tea ages more dynamically than any other tea type. The resulting aged tea is mellow and has a sweet taste and silky mouth-coat. Pu-erh teas are often classified by their year and region of production, much like wine vintages. The rarest pu-erh teas are made with tea leaves that are hand-harvested from wild and semi-wild antique tea trees (100 years and older). They continue to gain value with aging, and have been touted in the press as an investment tea. On an early tea-buying trip to China, I saw Japanese businessmen picking up pu-erh tea cakes from their personal tea lockers at a high-end purveyor's shop, like they were retrieving jewels from a safe deposit box. Compared with other teas, pu-erh has an almost cult-like following among tea lovers, and some people consider it a sacred relic of ancient tea cultures and traditions.

Only in recent years has good-quality pu-erh made its way into U.S. teahouses and retail shops. I drink organic loose leaf pu-erh, and the mini-bricks (*tuochas*) that are my travel teas of choice. There are also some excellent breakfast tea blends based on pu-erh. For special occasions, I'll bust out one of my well-hidden larger pu-erh bricks and chip away at it for guests. It always becomes the talk of the party.

By the way, the daughter who spat out her first sip of pu-erh into Boulder Creek at that seminar at the Dushanbe Teahouse now can't go a day without it. So if you haven't yet, next time you're in an adventurous mood, give pu-erh tea a try. Even if you don't fall for it at first sip, it just might develop into a healthy habit over time.

Pu-erh Tea

All pu-erh (POO-air) tea is made with sun-dried broad tea leaves from the Southern province of Yunnan, China, where the tea-growing season can last as long as eight or nine months each year. Pu-erh tea can be aged for many years. Because it continues to oxidize as it ages, Pu-erh can evolve and improve with age like a fine wine. It's often presented as a black tea, perhaps because of its dark red liquor, but it is in fact its own unique tea type. Pu-erh is higher in caffeine than black tea, yielding about 60 mg per 8-ounce (240-ml) serving. In both its fully oxidized and aged forms, it undergoes secondary oxidization caused by organisms that continue to develop in the tea, giving it strong antibacterial qualities (like blue cheese). The older the pu-erh, the more pricey it can be. Pu-erh tea comes in many different forms—from loose smaller-leaf tea, to large-leaf tea, larger tea bricks and tiny (coin-size) tea cakes.

According to traditional Chinese medicine, pu-erh tea has body-warming and potent digestive properties. Pu-erh is often consumed as a tea that dispels or cleanses the body of fat and toxins from meat and oily foods. Many people in Asia, where it is consumed as a detox tea, feel that pu-erh is the best cure for a hangover. In France, pu-erh is also widely popular and consumed by many women as a beauty and dieting tea. People go crazy for pu-erh tea as a weight loss solution in the U.S. because it's been shown to help enhance fat metabolism. It's this fat metabolizing mechanism that makes it a heart-healthy tea. Pu-erh tea bonds to cholesterol, retarding its absorption as it goes through the digestive tract, so the body doesn't absorb the fat and the arteries and veins are kept clean.

BULLETPROOF TEA RECIPE

Bulletproof Coffee and Bulletproof Tea are touted by fitness gurus and followers of Paleo diets to both satisfy and energize. These power drinks are rooted in traditional Tibetan butter tea, or *po cha*, a rich, brothy brew made from pu-erh, salt and yak butter. Butter tea has been a staple throughout many regions of the Himalayas for over a thousand years, where it's drunk throughout the day for its warming and energy-rich character. It helps provide sustenance for everyday living in the harsh, cold and arid conditions at high altitude. Many Westerners have been exposed to this tradition while traveling to Tibet, Nepal, Bhutan and India.

If you want to try this intriguing concoction without the expense of traveling halfway around the globe, you can simply use a few substitutions to make it yourself. Since it's likely impossible to find freshly churned yak butter at your local market, you can substitute organic butter from grassfed cows and virgin coconut oil, to give it the right consistency (and a lovely coconut aroma). Instead of using a traditional tall wooden churn, called a *cha dong*, to mix up your brew, a basic blender does a great job in a fraction of the time and is often what's used to make the drink today in Tibet. This is a modern rendition of butter tea you can make at home.

Modern Butter Tea

Yields one serving

1 cup (240 ml) strongly brewed pu-erh tea, or pu-erh tea blend (5 minute steep)

1 tsp (5 g) organic unsalted butter

1 tbsp (15 g) organic virgin coconut oil

A touch of honey (optional)

Put all the ingredients in a blender. Mix on high for one minute until frothy. (Use caution when opening the hot blender.)

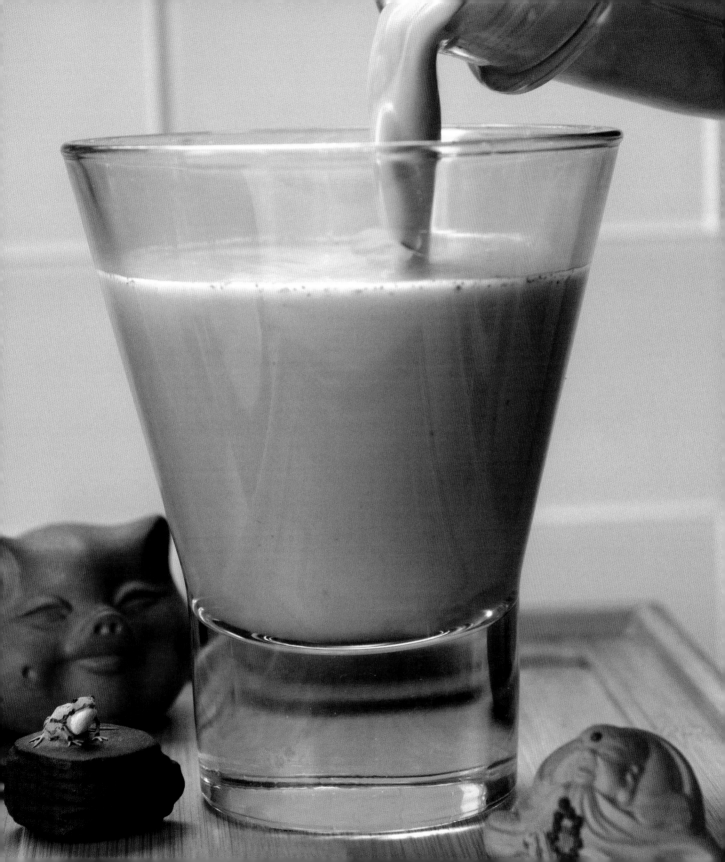

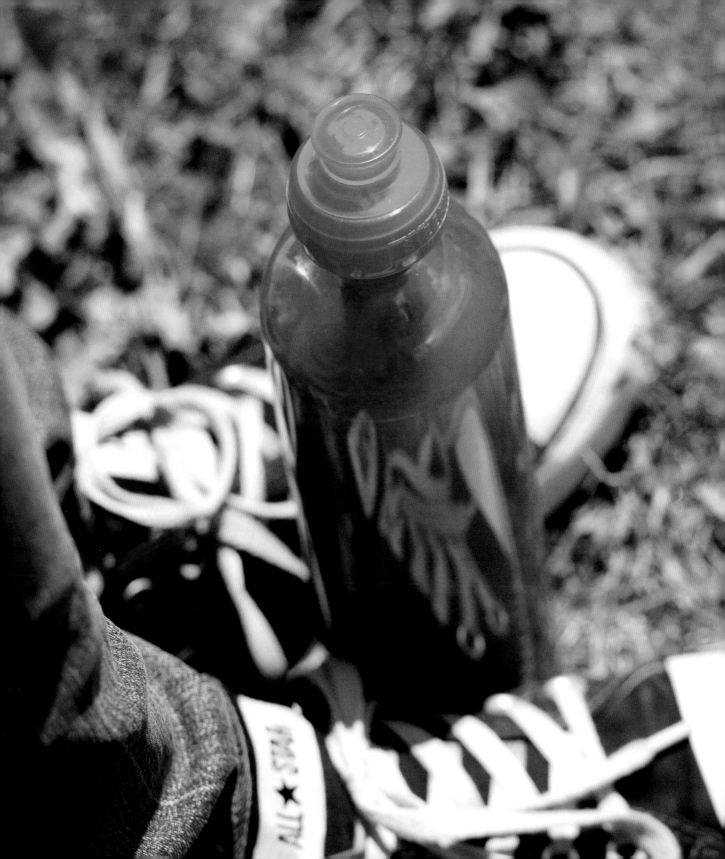

Chapter 6

CANCER HATES FITNESS

THERE'S NO ONE GIANT STEP—IT'S A LOT OF LITTLE STEPS

Cancer Climber

"You don't have to be the best, you just have to be your best." Sean Swarner is the first cancer survivor to summit Mount Everest. As a teen, he was diagnosed with two unrelated forms of cancer and was not expected to live. He did, however, and overcame both cancers. This inspirational athlete has only one functioning lung, but didn't see that as an obstacle to completing the IRONMAN World Championship in Hawaii and climbing the Seven Summits. He has become an author and motivational speaker, and founded The CancerClimber Association, where he shares his message and the message of other survivors of healing, hope and triumph with cancer patients and survivors worldwide through climbing and adventure-related challenges.

"Everyone's going to be diagnosed or affected by cancer in our lifetimes," says Swarner. "We only have one life, so it's time for people to take notice." Swarner says he thinks about his body's health and immunity on a microscopic level: "The body's just going to deteriorate from exposure to toxins through food and environment, if we don't take precautions." He says he eats everything in moderation and fortunately has always loved vegetables, which he feels are the most important component of a healthy diet. Fitness is another key component to his wellness, which he says is important on many levels. First off, it helps him stay in shape—this challenge seeker is currently training for a climb up Mt. Rainier, his annual fundraiser up Mt. Kilimanjaro and a North Pole Trek. "Fitness also supports the all-important mind-body connection," says Swarner. "It makes me feel better. So even when I'm super busy, I force myself to step away from the computer to take time out for a run. It's my time, I know I'm accomplishing something with it, and I take that time to visualize my day, and even to visualize where I want to be one year from now. If you focus on the end result, and make it real to yourself and real in your mind, nothing will ever stop you."

NOT LOOKING SO GOOD

The American Cancer Society estimates that one in of every five cancer deaths in the U.S. is linked to excess body weight, and the National Cancer Institute estimates this to be as high as 40 percent in the case of some cancers. In addition to its ability to store fat, adipose tissue (aka body fat) is a highly active hormonal and metabolic organ. As this adipose tissue expands, it creates chemical stimuli that increase the production of hormones whose job it is to regulate energy balance. This, in turn, can create chronic inflammation, which may directly promote cancer cell growth. Bottom Line: You don't want dysfunctional adipose tissue, which is what happens when it becomes too enlarged. What's more, obesity is also linked with a decrease in production of protective anti-inflammatory hormones. Double whammy.

Body Mass Index (BMI) is the relationship of weight to height determined by dividing a person's weight in kilograms (kg) by his or her height in meters squared. More weight at a lower height results in a higher BMI. A BMI of over 30 is considered obese. A projection from the National Institutes of Health estimates that if the current trends in obesity continue, that will contribute about 500,000 additional cases of cancer in the U.S. by 2030. The same analysis also made the point that if every U.S. adult reduced their BMI by one percent, this would reverse the trend and actually result in the avoidance of approximately 100,000 new cases of cancer. And get this—that one percent of BMI is just about 2 pounds (1 kg) per average adult.

BACK UP—HOW DID WE GET THIS WAY?

The American way of eating, which has now become the rich nations' way of eating, causes people to be hungry, malnourished and overfed, all at the same time. Twenty-first century bodies residing in successful economies tragically hunger for real food. Now how is that possible? For the most part, we don't lack for food in this country. Compared with the rest of the world, every last American is in the top 20 percent economically. But unfortunately, our national diet isn't nourishing, and many of the calories that make up part of our daily intake are highly addictive processed foods that are high in sugars, fats and chemicals with names we can't pronounce. One-third of the U.S. population is chronically obese, and one in four U.S. adults is affected by metabolic syndrome, which is a group of nasty risk factors including increased waist circumference, increased blood sugar levels, elevated triglycerides and increased blood pressure. Do you think this could all be coincidence? Probably not.

Our hunter-gatherer ancestors never knew where their next meal was going to come from. Because of the effort it took to get food to their mouths, each bite would have been savored as a precious morsel. But then, as agriculture developed in later civilizations, mankind could afford to become more sedentary. Modern supermarkets and mega shopping centers along with the transition to a car culture, drive-throughs, take-out and delivery brings this to our ridiculous current-day extreme: **Humans no longer need to move to eat**. And we never need to come into contact with any of the plants or animals that make up the food on our plates. Eric Schlosser, author of *Fast Food Nation*, says that about 90 percent of the average American's food budget is allocated toward processed foods. Our taste buds have been sucked into their super-intense flavors, and we're now a nation of junkies for fat, sugar, artificial flavorings and sodium. The truth is, when we don't prepare our own meals, we really know don't what's going onto our plates and into our mouths. And the more processed and addictive the foods we eat are, the more prone we are to just reaching for things to eat out of habit.

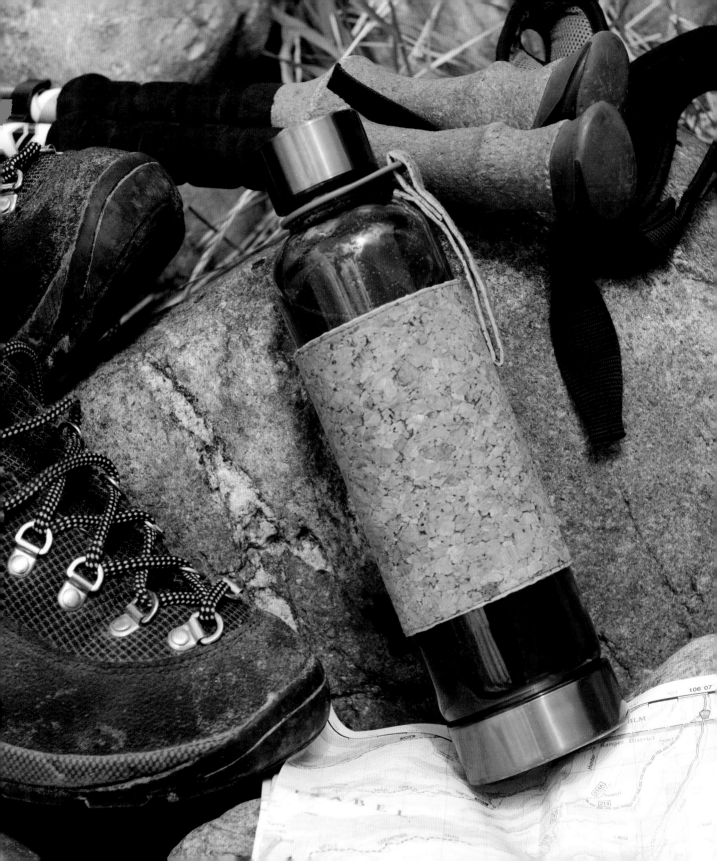

TEA WILL HELP YOU KEEP IT REAL

When you're just eating or drinking out of habit, you're probably not really savoring or enjoying your food. Hectic eating on the run, in your car or at your desk are perfect examples of simply fueling your body without pleasure or appreciation for food. This is such an easy routine to get into when we're busy, unfortunately. The subtle trick, which can seem impossible, is to change your relationship with food and start eating consciously. Nutritious food you cook yourself doesn't need to cost more money, but it does take time to make. It's really no different than taking the time to steep a perfect cup of tea for yourself. **Your new tea habit can be the perfect kick-starter for mindful eating.**

Weight management through tea drinking has been practiced for over 1,000 years. It's even described in the 8th century Chinese pharmacopoeia *Bencao Shiyi*, a practical guide for clinical diagnosis and prescriptions. And now, 1,300 years later, this practice is being validated by scientific research studies confirming the effect of tea catechins on helping to reduce body fat, but only if you have it to lose. One thing the findings indicate is that the decrease in excess body fat from tea catechins has been observed to be most substantial in subjects with a high Body Mass Index (BMI). So you won't be dropping from a size 6 to a size 4 in a hurry thanks to green tea, which is actually a good thing. Reducing unnecessary fat in people with an already low BMI would not be wellness-promoting. Tea just wants to help get you in the best possible physical shape.

THE SKINNY ON TEA & WEIGHT LOSS

Burn an extra 100 calories without lifting a finger or breaking a sweat? The promise of weight loss, not cancer prevention, is what gets most people in our country to buy green tea. Too bad for them, they probably missed the chapter on just how much good those canned and bottled teas really do for you or your waistline. But the fad really is based in a truth—tea actually helps boost your metabolic rate of burning calories. **It's the secret of the skinny.**

SIMPLY ADDING TEA TO YOUR DIET WILL HELP YOU LOSE WEIGHT: MYTH

Researchers have concluded that tea can be effective at boosting metabolism. Tea catechins increase your energy expenditure by helping turn fat into energy. This means that if you add green tea with no additives and zero calories to your routine, and keep everything else the same, you'll tip the calorie balance in your favor. But even downing 2 liters of green tea won't deal with burning through a daily pizza and fast-food burgers habit. Tea will help you, but it needs you to take the lead! If you're looking to reduce some unneeded fat from your frame, try this for just three days: Begin your 5 cups (1.2 L) a day tea habit, and try some new and healthy foods, choosing and eating mindfully. Variety is a key tip here, both in your teas and your nutrition because keeping things interesting helps spur more conscious eating. And of course, you'll help your weight loss along even more if the tea you drink is unsweetened.

TEA WILL ASSIST YOUR BODY IN INHIBITING THE PRODUCTION OF FAT CELLS: TRUTH

Tea has been shown to help reduce abdominal paunch by inhibiting your gut's ability to absorb dietary fats, thanks again to its catechins. That's right, tea catechins go for the layer around your middle, called visceral fat, first. Clinical studies have concluded that daily ingestion of 400 mg of tea catechins significantly decreases body fat. That's the equivalent of 5 cups (1.2 L) of white, green or oolong tea, brewed fresh. Fancy meeting you here, EGCg—this is the polyphenol which makes it all happen. When you drink a catechin-rich tea, the EGCg gets into the cells of your intestinal tract, where it disrupts the intestinal processes that lead to fat tissue formation in your belly. It does this by using its antioxidant mechanism again, this time forming complexes with lipids and enzymes, thus wreaking havoc with the critical steps involved in your body's absorption of dietary fat.

TEA PROVIDES A BOOST TO EXERCISE-INDUCED WEIGHT LOSS, FURTHER STIMULATING THE DESTRUCTION OF FAT THROUGH EXERCISE: TRUTH

One of the best ways to boost your burn when you work out is to drink 2 to 4 cups (480 to 960 ml) of tea half an hour before you exercise. Research suggests this can help your body to burn up to 17 percent more calories during moderately intense movement for up to three hours. The combination of tea catechin intake with consistent exercise sessions can increase overall energy expenditure more than the exercise alone would accomplish. What's more, consistent intake of tea catechins has been shown to maintain an increased metabolic rate and raise your daily calorie burn by about 4 percent. That doesn't sound like much, but over the course of a year, it can add up to more than 10 pounds (5 kg) on most adult frames. So go steep some catechin-heavy tea (white, green or oolong), take a brisk walk and feel good about what you're doing for your beautiful self.

TEA IS A NATURAL APPETITE SUPPRESSANT: TRUTH

A study by Swedish researchers found that unsweetened, caffeinated green tea was super effective in satiating your hunger. You guessed it: It's the EGCg, working overtime in your gut, boosting levels of cholecystokinin (CCK), a gastrointestinal hormone which tells your central nervous system when to say *basta* to your plate of pasta. Think of it as a home-grown hunger suppressant that induces a satiating effect. Subjects who were given green tea instead of water in the study were less likely to crave even their favorite foods for up to two hours after drinking the tea.

THE BOTTOM LINE

Tea can be used as a subtle, yet effective tool in helping you muster your willpower and give you a nice nudge toward your weight management goals. Sipping on a warm mug or cold glass of tea throughout the day won't get you to drop a dress size in three days, but it can help you get the long-term results that are more likely to stay with you. The bottom line if you're looking to drop some pounds is that you need to consistently create a calorie deficit by taking in less than you're burning. And keep in mind that wellness includes just enjoying yourself. Use that 80/20 rule from chapter 5 (page 82). Splurge when you feel the need to treat yourself, and most importantly, always cook, eat and steep with feelings of love and self-care.

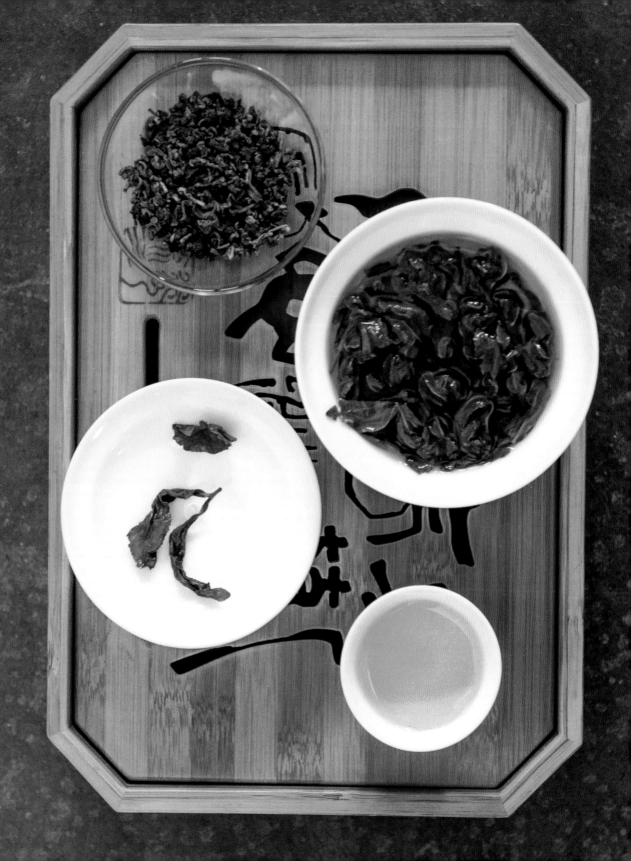

ABOUT OOLONG TEAS

Several studies have found that drinking oolong tea will help you metabolize a few percent more calories than green tea. The research points to a specific polymerized polyphenol in oolong tea, which works in combination with EGCg, creating an increase in energy expenditure. And losing weight never tasted so good. Oolong teas are truly unforgettable with their delicate, yet complex aromas and naturally fragrant flavors, which range from lilac and orange blossoms to smooth or smoky honey. Oolongs are varied and multifaceted in their flavor profiles. They boast the body and complexity of a black tea, with the brightness and freshness of a green tea.

A very favorite and desired tea amongst connoisseurs, oolongs hail from the Wuyi mountains in Fujian, China, as well as from Taiwan. From lightly oxidized to dark roasted, oolongs can be fragrantly floral to lusciously rich and sophisticated. Taiwan is famous for its many wonderful oolong teas, and deservedly so. In China, Teguanyin (Iron Goddess of Mercy) is one of the most famous oolong teas whose characteristic flavor comes from the charcoal used when firing the leaves after the oxidation process. This style of oolong is named for the Buddhist goddess of compassion. There are several versions of a legend dating back to the 18th century that tell of the softhearted goddess Guanyin helping a poor tea farmer discover the extraordinary tea plants and process which are now used to produce this tea.

It took me a long time to learn to appreciate oolong teas for their taste and changes in flavor profile between steeps. As Americans, I think we tend to choose consistency in our food and beverage products over the unknown, even if it holds some wonderful surprises in store for us. But from the very beginning, what I could appreciate was the consummate quality of the leaves and careful craftsmanship used to make these teas. Oolongs are laboriously handcrafted, truly a labor of love, and their price tags are rightly reflective of that. However, you more than make up your initial investment on them because oolong leaves can be infused multiple times. Each steep will unveil a new facet of its flavor profile. My favorite steeps are usually the second or the third, but some of the more complex oolongs continue augmenting in flavor through the fourth or fifth steep. You can make a half-gallon (2 L) pitcher of iced oolong by steeping the same teaspoonful of leaves 8 times, and your guests will swear they've never had a tea that tasted so good!

SKINNY TEAS AND HERBALS

Oolong teas are semi-oxidized, which places them between green and black teas in terms of oxidation and their mix of antioxidants. This spans a broad range, ranging from under 20 percent to as high as 80 percent. Many more lightly oxidized oolongs are rich in catechins, like green teas. They're often cited as one of the best teas for weight loss. Caffeine level is moderate.

Pu-erh teas have long been considered a health tea by the Chinese. In traditional Eastern medicine, pu-erh is believed to invigorate the spleen, counteract alcohol toxins (cure your hangover), release stomach heat and descend stomach chi (help keep you regular). Pu-erh has also been considered a weight loss supplement due to its ability to aid in fat metabolism. To give pu-erh the best opportunity to work its magic, the best time to drink it for weight management is an hour after finishing your meal. Caffeine level is high.

Green teas are what have stirred up the tea-for-weight-loss craze and spawned hundreds of new products, bottled, canned, powdered and otherwise, over the past decade. As always, your best bet for getting the max burn and the best bang for your buck is to brew your own. Adding lemon to your green tea for weight loss could make its flavor more appealing to you. In addition, the lemon also acts as a natural appetite suppressant. Caffeine level is moderate.

White teas can be considered the leading edge of catechin-rich teas for weight loss. They're subtle and delicate in flavor, and very easy to drink. They cold brew fabulously. Caffeine level is low.

Ginger is a root often recommended for helping improve circulation in the body. Spicy and comforting for digestion, ginger root has been used since ancient times as a natural digestive aid for relieving nausea, bloating and menstrual cramps, as well as eliminating intestinal gas. Caffeine-free.

Hibiscus is touted for its cleansing properties that help keep your circulatory system flowing and pumping. Since it's naturally caffeine-free, hibiscus is a great way to stay healthfully hydrated any time of day. It also offers a natural source of vitamin C. Cold brews like a champ. Caffeine-free.

Fennel seed is thought to be purifying and is an active herbal in many cleanse teas. Its naturally sweet flavor may work to curb your cravings. A known diuretic, it is helpful in relieving bloating. Caffeine-free.

Chamomile may have a positive influence on weight loss. This could be directly related to its ability to help relieve stress and induce a feeling of relaxation, both of which are important to supporting healthy weight management, as well as its ability to help stimulate the production of gastric juices. Caffeine-free.

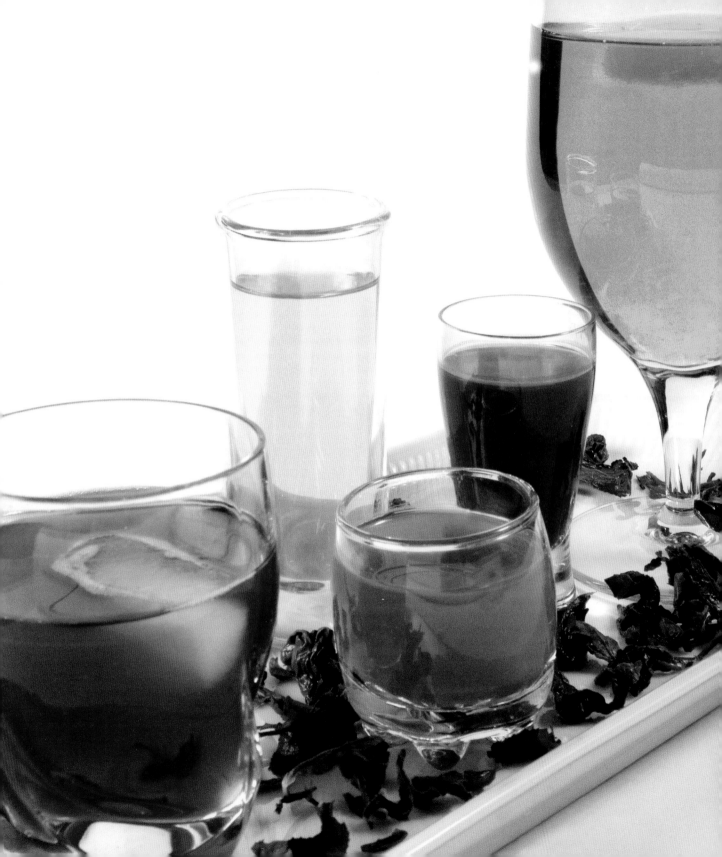

LOST AND FOUND—HOW I GOT MY BIKING PHYSIQUE BACK

Many of us have had this strange wake-up call—either getting on the scale at the doctor's office, or trying to put on an old favorite dress—that makes us truly wonder where those extra 10 or 20 pounds (5 or 10 kg) came from. What's ridiculous about it is that just like many other bad habits, taking on a bunch of extra pounds can happen without you even realizing it.

One spring I got out on my bike for the first time and couldn't understand what had happened to my bike geometry to get my knees to keep bumping into my stomach. This was the same bike I'd been riding for years, and it had always fit me. What was going on? As I pedaled on, I realized my gut was indeed getting in the way of my pedal stroke. Seriously??? So I started doing an inventory of what had changed in my life. Both my daughters had left for school, so I was living alone. I'd been really busy at work and often stayed at my office until 6:30 or 7 PM. When I felt a lull around 5:30 or 6, when previously I would have been home making dinner, I'd just grab whatever I could find to power me through the next hour, and then I'd go home and cook dinner. So what was that snack? It wasn't always unhealthy, either nuts and dried fruit or sometimes chips, and it probably averaged 300 to 350 calories a day. That adds up to about 7,000 calories a month, and I'd been doing this for about nine months to total 63,000 calories. If I hadn't made any other changes to my intake (diet) or calorie burn (activity level) that would amount to 18 pounds (8 kg). When I got off the bike, I went straight to our warehouse and got on the shipping scale. Up 17 pounds (7 kg). Wow. I'd been clueless, or in some serious denial. How could I not notice 17 pounds (7 kg)?! That was a gain of more than 12 percent. Whatever, now I was mad and ready to do something about it.

It's intimidating to break any habit, but I find that just three days of resetting my relationship with eating goes a very long way toward turning mindless munching into mindful eating. I've finally learned to admit that my biggest offenders are chips and bread. To break that craving, I just have to cut out any and all processed foods, breads, crusts, baked goods and chips. And I do the same for any added sugar. This may seem extreme, but truly, it's not nearly as obnoxious as it sounds. I still have oatmeal in the morning, and whole grain pasta or brown rice with my dinner, so I'm not without carbs. But I know that bread has just enough sugar in it to get my appetite roaring. And after three days of making friends again with simpler meals, minus all my offenders, I can take a big sigh and just eat what I decide I want, and not what my body had gotten wired to tremble and jump to have me grab.

My personal little secret to kick this process off is that I buy a super special green tea as my new treat. I'll always try to find one that I've not yet had before. Each morning of the three days of this reset, I'll brew up an insulated growler jug full, and sip a ridiculously excellent cup of green tea every half hour throughout the day. This keeps my body from screaming at me. After three days, I'm able to regain control and keep plugging away with conscious choices. I don't have to deny myself a glass of red wine with dinner or the occasional piece of dark chocolate. So what's the moral to this story? After doing this and cycling daily for 3 months, those 17 pounds (7 kg) were GONE, and I was BACK.

TEAS FOR BOOSTING FITNESS

Getting fit and strong usually comes with the pleasant by-product of managing obesity. So put climbing Mount Everest back on your bucket list, because tea will give you the gusto you need to summit not only your daily workout but your biggest dreams. And here's a bonus: Strong is the new pretty. Intense or prolonged exercise can produce considerable amounts of oxidative stress, and at times, either from fatigue or overtraining, the human body's natural oxidant defense system isn't powerful enough to restore the damage. Thus, the argument goes, athletes need to accelerate their intake of antioxidants. Observers of the athletic scene sometimes wonder if it's more than a coincidence that the best endurance athletes in the world, Kenyan runners, sip hot black tea throughout the day. So is tea a near-perfect sports drink? If a couple of cups of tea are consumed about an hour before exercise, the caffeine content is likely to enhance performance in high-intensity athletic events. When tea is consumed post-exercise, its rich antioxidant content may well boost recovery and limit oxidative stress to muscles. It's true that more research is needed in this area, but our present state of knowledge suggests that all tea types are an attractive drink for both endurance and sprint athletes.

Black teas provide an energizing effect from caffeine. But more interestingly, findings show that the theaflavins in black tea may lead to an improved recovery rate and a reduction in oxidative stress responses following intense exercise, which facilitates more frequent workouts. Moderate to high caffeine, 40 to 60 mg per 8-ounce (240-ml) serving.

Green teas are rapidly becoming a beverage of choice amongst many endurance athletes. Among the many touted health benefits of green tea is the boost it can provide for increasing mental focus, as well as increasing endurance. Low to moderate caffeine, 15 to 30 mg per 8-ounce (240-ml) serving.

Roasted green teas are extremely low in tannins, high in antioxidants and super easy on the stomach with great flavor and a robust sense of nourishment. Low caffeine, 10 to 20 mg per 8-ounce (240-ml) serving.

ABOUT CHAI

Your first sip of chai will conjure up images of warm and colorful spice markets. As the masala (spice mix) profile reveals itself to your senses, you'll find yourself sensuously warmed from the inside out. This fragrant mug is a potent blend of different ayurvedic herbs and black tea. Chai originated over 5,000 years ago in south Asia, when it was created as a healing ayurvedic warming tonic and digestive aid, originally without tea. With the advent of British tea plantations in India in the 19th century, tea was added to the spicy beverage. The black tea base of chai is almost always Assam. Every family in India has their own proprietary recipe for the chai masala using green cardamom, cinnamon, ginger, pepper and fennel. In neighboring mountain regions, sherpa families blend masala chai not only to warm and energize, but to be physically assistive in the higher Himalayas, thanks to the addition of elements which help with adjustment to altitude. These high altitude chais might have herbs such as tulsi holy basil, ginseng, ginkgo biloba and schizandra. Chai is traditionally served as a sweetened black tea mixed with milk and the chai masala.

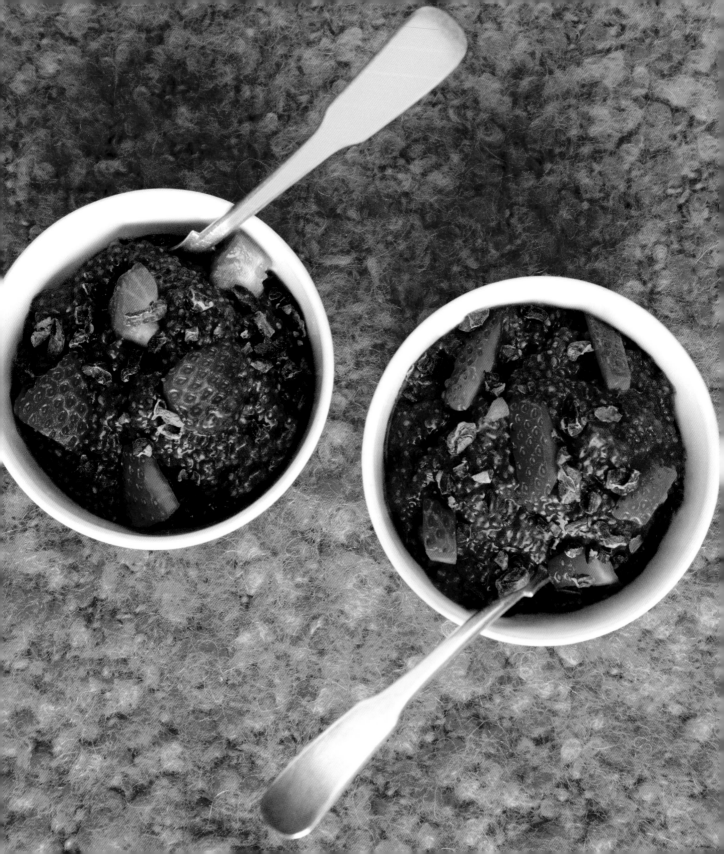

Cocoa Chai Chia Seed Breakfast Bowl

For a delicious fitness-boosting start to your morning, try this easy refrigerator breakfast bowl.

Yields two servings

1 cup (240 ml) strong brewed chai tea

4 tbsp (40 g) chia seeds

1 tbsp (11 g) cacao nibs

1 tbsp (7 g) cocoa powder

6 tbsp (89 ml) almond milk (or non-dairy milk of choice)

1–2 tsp (5–10 ml) maple syrup, or sweetener to taste (optional)

Sliced fruit and/or berries, for topping

Mix all the ingredients together, cover and let chill and set overnight. Divide and spoon into two bowls. Serve with sliced fruit and berries.

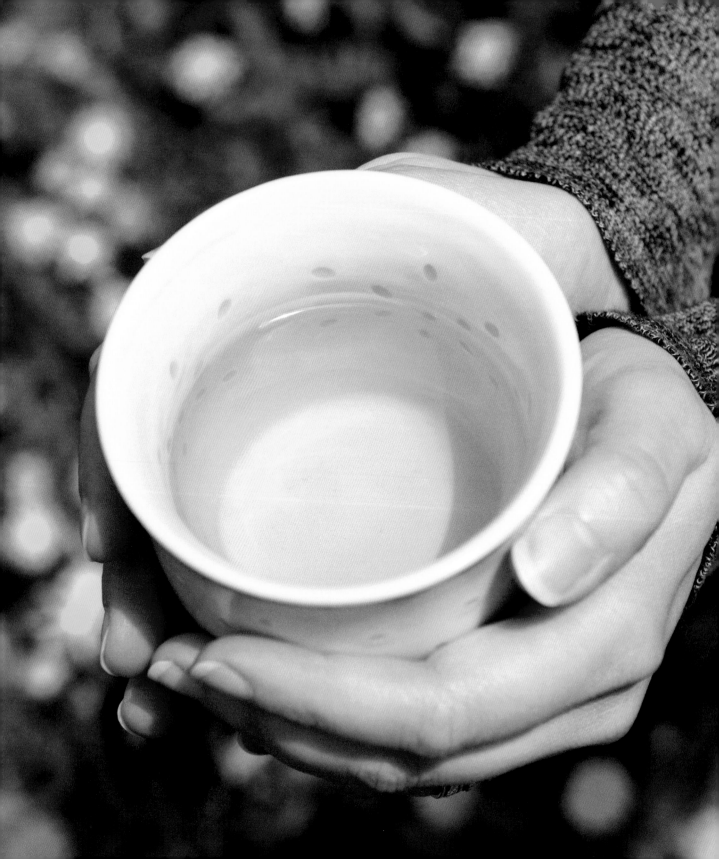

Chapter 7

CANCER HATES OM TIME

DROP AND GIVE ME ZEN

Cowgirls vs. Cancer

"Self-care is non-negotiable," insists Margaret Burns-Vap, founder of Big Sky Yoga Retreats. "We have the chance to learn something new every day that can improve our health and wellness and therefore help everyone we touch in our lives. It's not selfish. And a lot of women don't do this because they feel guilty!" The former cosmetics industry exec-turned yogini entrepreneur teaches women that self-care is not a luxury. "You need to do it. Take advantage of every opportunity to improve your situation and your health and better enjoy your time on this planet." I experienced this first-hand for myself on one of her Winter Wellness yoga retreats, which is where I did my very first tea meditation led by Margaret herself. For me, the combination of tea, meditation and yoga, in beautiful Montana nature, away from home and the office was pure bliss. This is the essence of her mantra "Yeehaw and Namaste."

In 2010, Margaret added cancer-kicking scholarships to her internationally acclaimed yoga retreat business. "It seemed that whenever we turned around, we were hearing about a new case of cancer hitting a friend or family member, and I just started thinking, what can I do about this to make a positive impact and give back?" She started fundraising and offering scholarships for breast cancer fighters on her women-only retreats. Now eight to ten ladies come together for an exclusive annual Cowgirls vs. Cancer retreat. Participants are chosen through a thoughtful nomination process where they have to address what horses and yoga, and "Yeehaw and Namaste" mean to them. Many of them already knew that yoga can be an important health tool in their recovery. Burns-Vap was herself amazed at the empowering bonding experience she saw in women from being with others with whom they share a lot of common ground. "This retreat hits home the message of the importance of self-care. At Cowgirls vs. Cancer, the alchemy of the powerful healing effect from the combination of yoga and horses is simply incredible."

THINK LESS. LIVE MORE.

Breathe deep, steep and sip, get your tea drinking pinky and your butt up in the air now. Tea, with meditation and yoga, can get you right there. Cancer downright hates this. Yup, cancer's totally bullied by you blissfully chanting om in a room with thirty other sweaty people doing yoga.

Let me fill you in on something—it took me years to figure out yoga. It's not about the poses. It's all about getting you out of your brain and into your heart. Your yoga instructors put you through what might seem like some ridiculous moves to help get you there. But when you start focusing 100 percent on relaxing while getting your butt way up in the air, your back splayed forward, and your head hanging down between your legs, there's not much room for anything outside the present moment—you are now nowhere but right here. As circuitous a route as it may seem, doing things such as getting into the perfect downward-facing dog, mountain biking down a treacherous ridge or playing a piece of music with friends are all legitimate ways to get to Om Time because your entire being is not concerned with time, and there's nothing left but the present moment. So what's up with the present moment that makes it so special? It's that you've had to shed all your stress to get there.

HOUSTON, WE HAVE A PROBLEM

Face it. So-called Modern-Day society is just one big mother-honking pressure cooker. **Stress is a legendary killer and a great cheerleader for cancer.** There's strong evidence linking chronic stress and cancer progression. The various mechanisms by which this takes place have been researched in hundreds of studies over the past several decades. Back up for a moment, you remember about free radicals, right? Stress causes your body to release more free radicals, sometimes more than your immune system can wipe up on a daily basis. What's know as the fight-or-flight response activates signaling pathways and induces chemical secretions of molecules, including the stress hormone cortisol, which undermines your health by suppressing immune function.

But there's a difference between short-lived stress, such as getting a speeding ticket, and repetitive or long-term chronic stress that you can't easily get away from, such as going to a job you hate every day or dealing with illness, death or divorce. Chronic stress works in complex ways. It triggers a domino effect of signals in the central nervous system which overwhelm the immune cells to the point where they can give up the fight, making the body more susceptible to the enemy. Yet another nasty mechanism of stress is the activation of a master gene called ATF3 (Activating Transcription Factor 3) that actually helps cells adapt to chronic stress. This gene has been identified as a critical enabler to the movement of cancer cells throughout the body. The body's overall reaction to stress gives cancer a friendly boost.

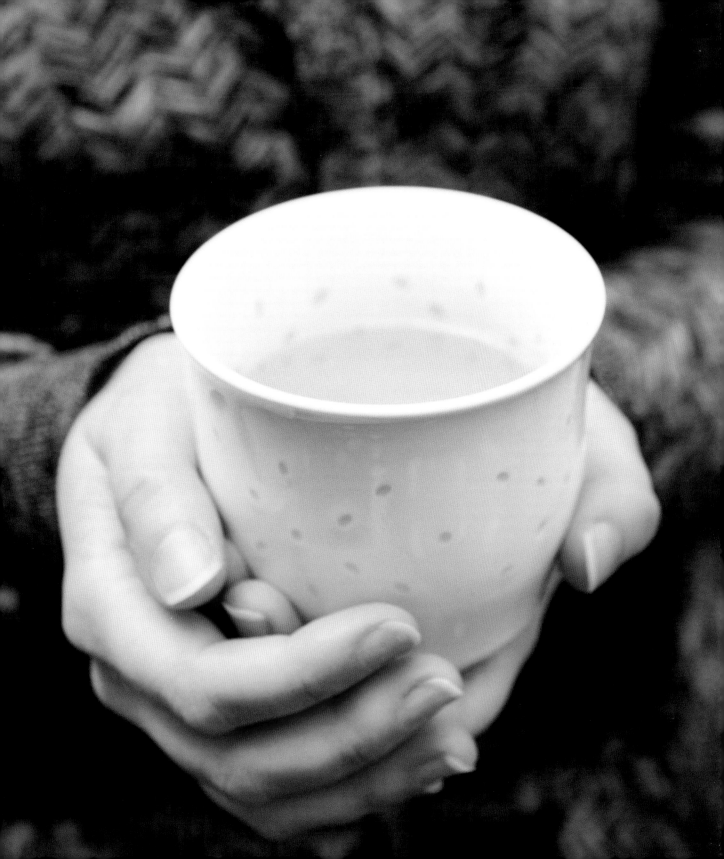

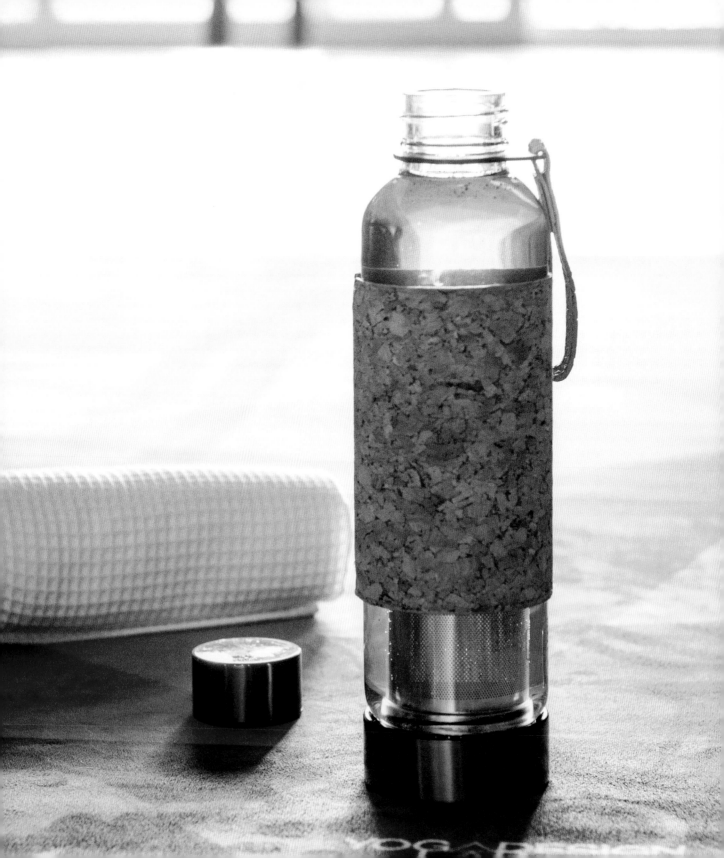

BE HERE NOW

Yoga and meditation work like detox for the brain. Their practice is a great way to find the courage to be vulnerable enough to get deep within yourself, to where the past is just a memory, the future is just a thought and there is only THE NOW. Yoga and meditation are both tools to help you get there, the every-minute, the present moment. Getting there isn't always easy, and many of us may never fully arrive at this point of zero stress. But no matter where you are with the yoga and meditation practice, you can become less stressed by listening more closely to your body. An easy way to get started with this is to focus only on your breath. If you can succeed in doing just that, breathing, you may be surprised at how amazing it feels to have nothing else to think about. When you manage to get yourself into the present moment, there's no space left between you and your innermost self. And when you get close to releasing absolutely everything else, and connecting with your innermost wild thing, you may just find pure, unbridled joy.

Sound ridiculous? Just try breathing mindfully like this:

* Sit anywhere—at your desk, in your car, on the floor.
* Start breathing slowly, fully, through your nose.
* Start counting your breaths.
* Focus for ten breaths on the intake.
* For the next ten, focus on breathing out.
* For the next ten, focus on breathing in through your right nostril.
* For the next ten, focus on breathing in through your left nostril.
* For the next ten, focus on having your breath fill your chest cavity.
* For the next ten, focus on having your breath fill your arms all the way down to your fingertips.
* For the next ten, focus on having your breath fill your legs all the way down to your toes.
* For the next ten, focus on having your breath fill you all the way down to your fingertips and toes.
* For the next ten, focus on having your breath fill your head. When you breathe in, imagine white and gold colors.
* For the last ten, focus on taking slower breaths and having them envelop your heart.
* Namaste. You've just completed a mindfulness meditation.

TEA AS STRESS BUSTER

A study of adults, previously not meditators, were trained to practice mindfulness meditation at home for 45 minutes each day. After eight weeks of practice they took 76 percent fewer sick days due to colds and influenza. Could it be that their immune systems were now totally able to handle the workload due to lower stress? Connecting with your breath is one of the few things you can do for your health that is even cheaper than tea.

Can you guess where we're headed with this? **Tea can also help soothe your stress.** This probably doesn't come as a surprise, because people have been offered a cuppa to make them feel better for centuries. Your grandma and the wizards in Harry Potter didn't need to read the studies to know that tea may speed up your recovery from the daily stresses in life. It does this several ways, in fact.

WE GOT THIS

One study found that people who drank black tea were able to de-stress faster than those who drank a fake tea substitute. All 75 study subjects were adult men. They had to give up all their usual caffeinated beverages. One group was given regular black tea and the other group was given a tea-free beverage which looked, smelled and tasted like black tea—so they all thought they were drinking real tea. All the participants drank their tea four times a day for six weeks, during which time they were monitored. The study found that the tea drinkers had lower levels of cortisol, the stress hormone, one hour after being faced with a stressful task. The task was that they had to defend themselves verbally in front of a video camera, after being threatened with losing their jobs or being accused of shop-lifting. What's interesting about the results in this study is that both groups experienced the same spikes in heart rate, blood pressure and hormone levels when faced with the unpleasant situation, but the tea drinking group came back to their baseline faster, and they reported feeling more relaxed. Cortisol levels dropped almost twice as much in the tea drinkers within 50 minutes of the stressful event. The black tea drinking group also had lower platelet activation, a marker for heart attack risk.

Remember that amino acid theanine? It's like a mash-up of chill pill with brain juice. Theanine allows tea to help you relax and focus at the same time. It occurs naturally in tea and is a relaxing agent that doesn't put you to sleep. First, this amino acid promotes alpha brain wave production, inducing a state of deep relaxation and mental alertness, much like the one you achieve when in a deep state of meditation. In combination with caffeine, it's especially clever in how it acts on some critical pathways in the brain. This molecule neutralizes the jittery and edgy effects of caffeine without affecting the mind-focusing aspects. Have you ever noticed that your body reacts differently to the caffeine in tea versus coffee? Theanine increases levels of dopamine. Dopamine is involved in many complex and critical neurological functions, including the regulation of cognition and attention. The other thing theanine does is increase the levels of the neurotransmitter GABA (Gamma-Amino Butyric Acid) in your brain. GABA works like the regulator that ratchets down the activity of the nerve cells responsible for your stress, fear and anxiety. And if that's not enough, theanine has been shown to clinically lower blood pressure.

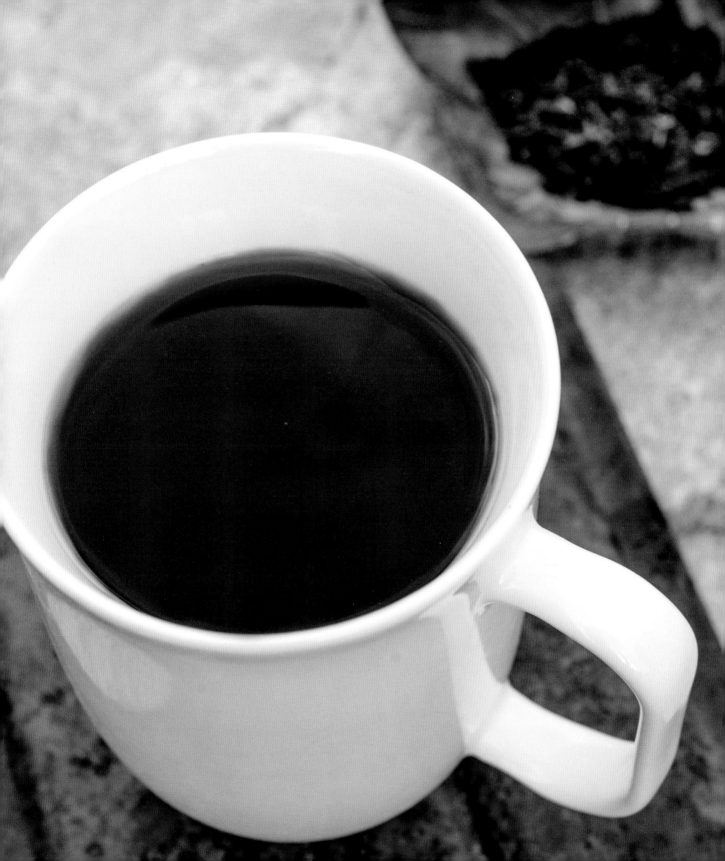

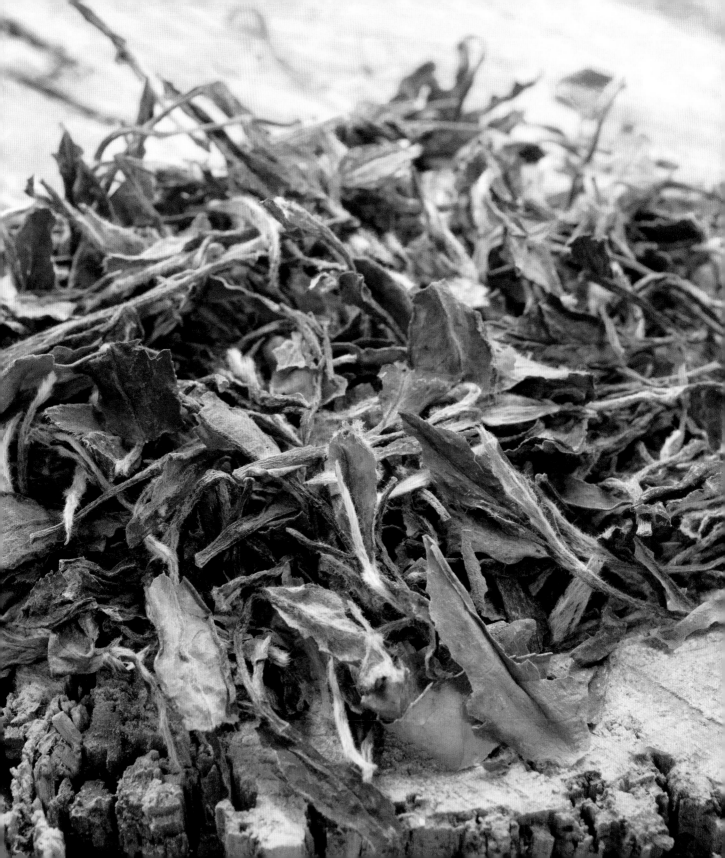

It's complicated, but once you dig down, it all begins to make sense as to why tea is often used to help support meditation. **Drinking tea has some of the same chemical and neurological effects as going into a deep meditative state.** This is a marriage made in Heaven, or Nirvana, in this case. Don't let stress get you down! This is even easier than weight management. One last tip: You'll be in the express lane to Zen if you reduce your coffee and alcohol consumption while increasing your tea intake.

ABOUT WHITE TEA

White tea is the most delicate tea in flavor and aroma, as the leaves are not rolled or crushed in the processing. They retain a silky, downy peach fuzz quality in the leaves. Because of the large, light leaves, white tea requires less tea by weight per serving. So it yields the least amount of caffeine of all teas, generally ranging from 5 to 10 mg per 8-ounce (240-ml) cup. This is one of the reasons why white tea is ideal for meditation. It can help you relax while focusing peacefully on tasks. Historically, Zen Buddhist monks have used this tea when they needed to stay quietly alert for long meditations. White tea is considered cooling, or anti-inflammatory, in Chinese medicine, and it's loaded with catechin polyphenols.

White tea was the favorite of the famous Tea Emperor in the 1100s. He was so preoccupied with his love of tea and his pursuit of the perfect cup that he lost his empire to invading Mongols. White teas have since traditionally been used as a tribute tea to the Chinese Emperor. When you first drink white tea, it seems quite tasteless, as if you were simply drinking hot water. However, after a while, you'll become aware of a subtle change in your breath and at the back of your mouth. It's almost as if you need to hone your senses more sharply to get to its heart. Instead of having a solid, dominant aroma like other types of tea, white teas tend to have a much more subtle, lingering fragrance. It's like when you take a deep breath in autumn, but can still sense a touch of summer in the air; or when you play a musical instrument, suddenly stop and for a long moment feel the music continuing, as if it were haunting the space. The Chinese refer to this subtle feel as "the taste between your teeth."

I've been blown away by the soothing, calming and uplifting practice of steeping and sipping this most subtle of teas. If I catch myself getting worked up, I'll take a breather and just to go through the ritual of making myself some fresh white tea and sit sipping a nice, delicate brew until all is once again right in my world. This tea works to refresh and quiet at the same time. I've made it my late afternoon new best friend—an easy obsession!

Most white teas are grown in the hilly coastal province of Fujian, China, where there are many exquisite and organic varieties of this tea type available today. The best known of these are Silver Needle (*Bai Hao Yin Zhen*) and White Peony (*Bai Mu Dan*). Fujian's climate is ideal for tea cultivation, which thrives in humidity and altitude. Fujian Province is 80 percent mountain, 10 percent water and 10 percent tea farms.

Doing yoga in the morning is like getting a natural dose of caffeine. It invigorates your body and can help you bring your morning caffeine intake down. After yoga, your body is rejuvenated and your mind is relaxed. You're at peace, while feeling energized, so you're not craving a big caffeine boost. Sipping on tea after doing yoga or meditation will prolong the benefits of stress reduction you achieved in your practice for a longer period into your day. Its relaxing effects will also help ease your transition back into a more chaotic environment.

Similarly, at night, you can yoga your way to better zzzz's. The practice is different in each case, as you might guess. A morning practice could have more upward swinging movements, such as Sun Salutations and big backbends which will make you feel like you're taking a shot of espresso. Morning practices tend to flow at an advancing pace. Evening practices might have longer, slower movements, many of which could be on the ground, easing your body into soothing stretches and relaxing back flattening poses.

Tea and yoga fuel a modern-day return to ancient roots through ritual. The tea culture represents a contrasting approach to the 21st century café scene. If coffee is the brew of efficiency and overstimulation, tea is the elixir that energizes and vitalizes by getting you to consciously press the pause button. Tea encourages reflection and offers reprieve. Some tea businesses hold workshops on healing and spirituality, while others even transform their daytime tea lounges into yoga studios by night. Similarly, yoga represents a different approach to modern workout culture. If the gym and the fitness craze represents going all out and over the top, yoga energizes and restores by getting you to consciously press the reset button. It nurtures inner strength, focus and awareness, as opposed to the no-pain-no-gain fitness approach. Both tea and yoga also share strong components of connection with one's self.

The Japanese tea ceremony Way of Tea originated as a form of Zen meditation. It is the art of finding beauty in every thing, no matter how small. The harmonious and tranquil experience of sensing stillness and living is shared in the moment between two people. A bowl of delicious pure green matcha is prepared by one person and received by another in a spirit of mutual understanding, grace, beauty and etiquette. The ceremony is meant to remind both the host and the guest of the uniqueness and impermanence of the present moment. Doing a tea ceremony or tea meditation before or after yoga is a beautiful and easy way to cultivate your health and wellness. Let go of trying to figure out the how and jump ahead to just doing it. Focus. Be present with where you are today, not yesterday. Learn to be patient with yourself. Remember that in meditation, as in yoga and in life, you can always go deeper on the exhale. And tell cancer to stay away from your Namaste space.

TEAS FOR OM TIME

White teas have become my personal favorite for meditation, or even for meditative activities such as journaling or just taking time out to think. Either hot or cold brewed, depending on the climate and your mood, they can help set you on the path to your meditative zone.

Green teas are an excellent all-around choice for morning yoga and meditation. For yoga, in particular, given the physical aspect of the poses, green tea is ideal as both a pre-practice energizer and post-practice restorative beverage. If you're drinking your pre-yoga tea on an empty stomach, roasted green tea or genmaicha are nice and easy on your tummy. Cold brewing makes them even smoother. Post-practice, there are a slew of great green choices, including dragonwell, sencha, clouds & mist and green jasmine tea. Green tea blends, as well as herbals, are a fun choice to cold brew for restoring and rehydrating after yoga.

Matcha A nice bowl of matcha or a matcha latte feels super nourishing after meditating. It's a ton less frustrating to whisk that puppy up when you're still centered and not running through your to-do list for the day.

Pu-erh teas are a great go-to before meditating or heading to yoga on those days when you feel like you might need a little extra help. We've all been there—the mornings when you either didn't sleep well enough or didn't eat right the night before. It's tough to empty your mind when you're not feeling it! The bold kick you get from pu-erh can get you there. A big hot brewed mug is my favorite way to go on those days.

Hot herbal teas often have a wonderful aromatic quality, which you'll appreciate all the more after opening your breathing during practice. They'll help gently cool you down as your body releases heat post-practice. They're also a great choice to rehydrate your body, which is important before you wind up your day for rest. Following a morning practice you can get feeling invigorated by herbal blends with lavender, mint and ginseng. Herbals with hibiscus, rose and chamomile will be more calming. Ginger and licorice are nice detoxifying choices for the evening.

Chai Traditional yogic tea is an Indian masala chai. This has an invigorating black Assam tea base spiced with chai masala: cinnamon, ginger, green cardamom, black pepper and perhaps cloves, fennel and/or star anise. Chai is prepared with hot simmering milk, and usually sweetened.

HOW TO DO A TEA MEDITATION

The act of steeping yourself a cup of tea is, in itself, already a meditative process. It's simple, routine in its steps and demands your attention. In selecting the tea leaves you wish to brew and the vessel you're going to brew them with, in getting the water to right temperature, in adding the correct proportions of tea leaves and water and in waiting for your infusion to get to the perfect point to drink, you're making your own personal tea ritual. The granddaddy of the Japanese Way of Tea Rikyu said, "The art of the Way of Tea consists simply of boiling water, preparing tea, and drinking it." Easy as 1-2-3, and profoundly nourishing. You can experience yet a whole new facet of tea by doing a simple tea meditation once the steeping is finished. It's a way to get to a much deeper appreciation for the spirit of tea and for healthful elixir you've just taken the care to offer yourself. Vietnamese Zen Master Thich Nhat Hanh summed it up when he said, "Peace, happiness and joy is possible during the time I drink my tea."

1. Choose a smallish tea cup you love which is easy and comfortable to hold in your hands. Prepare one of your favorite teas in it, mindfully. Stay with this. Don't multi-task.

2. Find a place you can sit comfortably and quietly, either in a chair or on the ground. Feel your sitz bones. Sit as straight as you are able to. (You'll breathe and sip better!)

3. Place your tea cup in front of yourself deliberately and respectfully. (Saucer or tray are optional.)

4. Take a moment to observe the tea in the cup. Note its color, and how it fills the cup. Admire it. Think about and acknowledge the journey it took to get this tea here from the tea plant, through the hands of the tea pluckers, over the ocean and to the ceremony of you preparing this drink. Give thanks for this cup of tea, and for this moment. Sit and stay with it for a minute.

5. Close your eyes. Reach for the cup of tea and feel its shape and texture. Feel the warmth of the cup with the tea in it. Imagine its weight when you'll pick it up.

6. Now pick up the cup, keeping your eyes closed. Feel the weight of the cup of tea in your hands. Feel that weight up your arms and into your body.

7. Bring the cup up to your face. Sense the warmth and the aroma of the tea with your eyes still closed. Stay and enjoy for a few breaths.

8. Bring the cup up to your mouth. See yourself as if you're watching from outside your own body. Feel the edge of the cup against your lips, sensing the shape of it. Take in the powerful aroma of the tea more deeply. Tilt the cup toward you in preparation for taking the first sip.

9. Take your first sip of the tea . . . you got it: M-I-N-D-F-U-L-L-Y. Take it SLOW. Continue, sip by sip. Experience every one, sensing their differences. Take a couple of slow breaths between each taste. Feel and savor the tea in your mouth, on your tongue, on your teeth. Where do you taste it the most? Feel it going down your throat. Try to sense where in your body you feel the benefits of drinking the tea. Breathe.

10. Place the cup back down in its original spot. Feel the effects of having sipped the tea on your palate. Breathe slowly. Feel the effects of the tea on your body. Open your eyes. Feel the effects of having sipped and swallowed the tea once again. Breathe deeply. Namaste.

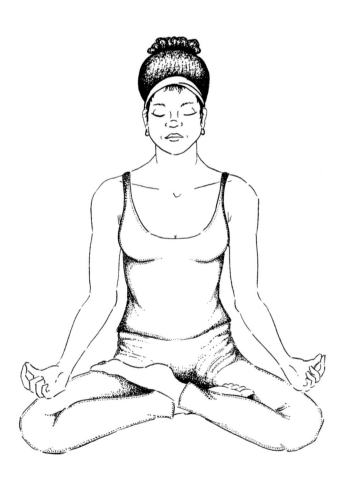

Meditation Tea Blends

The natural aromas of pure teas are exquisite, and doing a tea meditation with a favorite tea will surely give you a greater appreciation of that tea's qualities. Sometimes, it's nice to add even more of a lifting quality to your tea when you're meditating with it. These formulas are my three favorite blends for getting to a higher zen zone with tea.

Yield: 8 ounce (240 ml) serving

1 rounded tsp (1 g) white tea leaves

¼ tsp rose petals

Steep for 3 minutes using 175°F (80°C) water.

1 level tsp (2 g) green tea leaves

¼ tsp dried lavender, or 1 inch (2.5 cm) sprig fresh lavender

Steep for 3 minutes using 175°F (80°C) water.

1 level tsp (2 g) black tea leaves

One pinch dried peppermint or 1 fresh mint leaf

Steep for 5 minutes using boiling water.

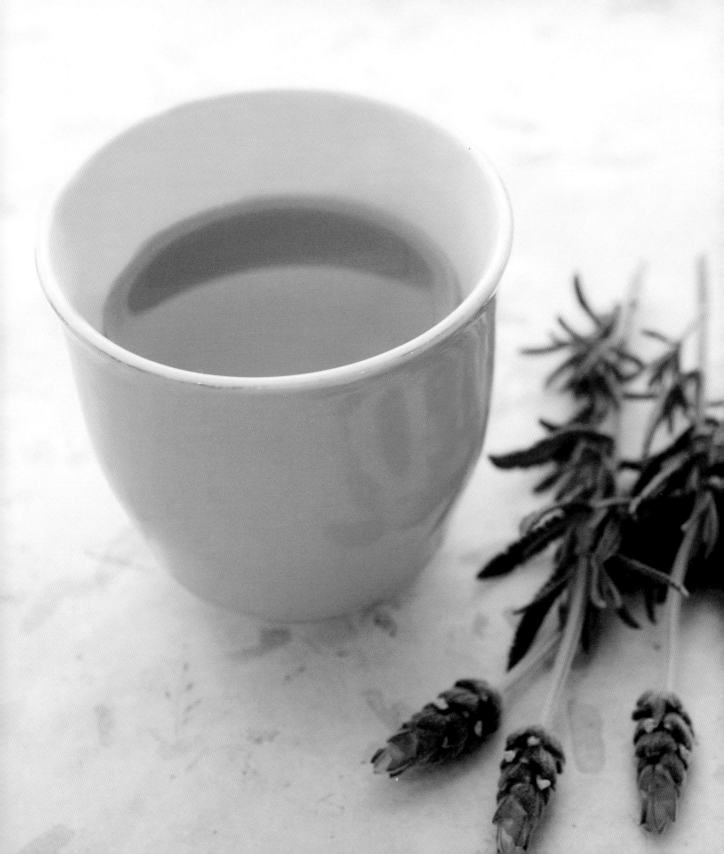

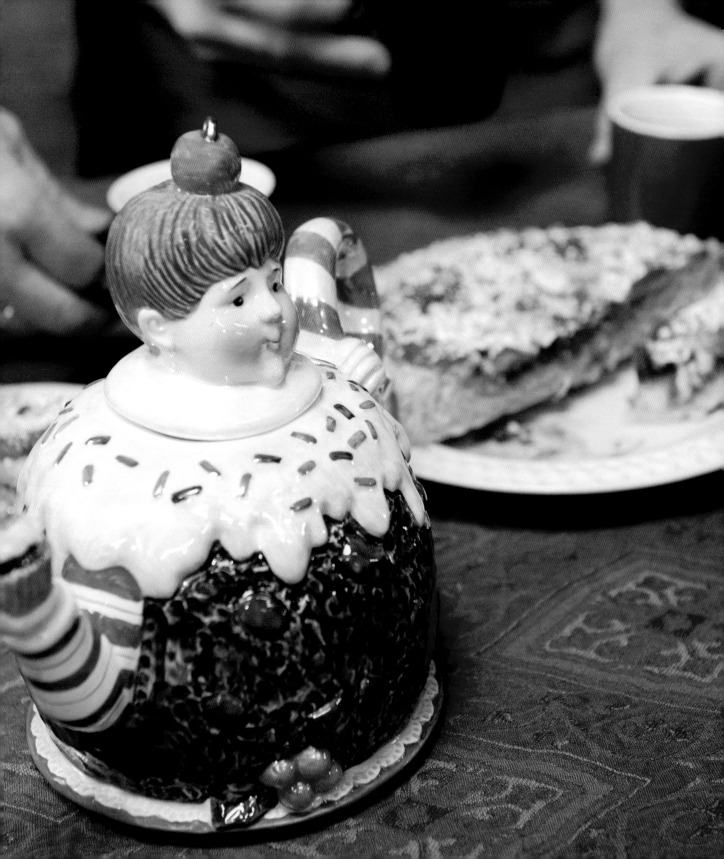

Chapter 8

CANCER HATES A PARTY

TRUE WEALTH IS SOMETHING MONEY CAN'T BUY

Living Journeys

Living Journeys Community Cancer Support, based in Colorado's Gunnison Valley, provides support and enrichment programs to families to help manage the fear, anxiety and confusion that often accompany a cancer diagnosis. The group's Executive Director, Darcie Perkins, said she was initially attracted to the group when she did their half marathon fundraiser. "I immediately realized how an organization such as this would have made a great difference to me when I was dealing with my cancer experience," said Perkins. "One of the critical issues that comes up when people have to all of a sudden manage everything that comes with facing cancer head on is financial stress. At Living Journeys, the money we raise goes to help bridge the gap when those situations become desperate, so patients can take the time to focus on themselves."

Patients who feel supported and calm enjoy an improved quality of life, which can in turn enhance their chances for positive treatment results. Living Journeys looks to bring emotional support into cancer patients' lives through group therapy sessions, offered several times a month, as well as grants for private therapy sessions, when necessary. Their enrichment programs include youth groups for kids who need help when family members are affected by cancer. Perkins explained that, "People don't realize the impact cancer has on all the family members. Kids process things differently. We partner with an adaptive sports program and professional therapists, who manage and run the activities, and provide emotional guidance. We lead an adventure day once a month, with activities ranging from skiing and ice climbing to horseback riding and hiking. These days out offer an outlet to focus on something way outside the sphere of fear, anxiety and stress of cancer."

Living Journeys is also part of the Community Wellness Program at the local hospital. "Even in our small, outdoorsy mountain community, we're not benign to cancer," says Perkins, "so raising awareness about the role nutrition plays in disease prevention and management is key."

WHAT ARE FRIENDS FOR?

Cancer doesn't want you out socializing and having fun. Cancer has a harder fight to face when you're with people you love, because they give you the strength and the power to fight back. Turns out you and your tea polyphenols are not the only warriors you've got in this fight. Several large-scale studies have examined the impact of social support and relationship satisfaction in cancer management, and the evidence indicates that high levels of social support are linked to improved clinical outcomes in cancer patients. Social support, in this case, is a reflection of an individual's sense of satisfaction in his or her personal relationships. An individual's sense of happiness in close personal and social relationships has the capacity not only to help his or her odds in fighting cancer but also to buffer actual physiological stress factors identified as risk factors for cancer. Those stress factors affect the biology of specific cellular and molecular signaling pathways that studies have identified can impact cancer growth and metastasis.

In a recent study on the topic, researchers followed more than 14,000 participants, surveyed at various stages in life about the nature of their social relationships. Information such as numbers of friends, marital status, religious affiliation and involvement in community domains, as well as whether they found their friends and relatives were critical, supportive, loving, argumentative or annoying was correlated against data on the participants' physical well-being. The researchers looked at four specific health markers: blood pressure, body mass index, waist circumference and a particular protein which measures inflammation, all key indicators of chronic daily stress which is known to have a link with the progression of disease. The wealth of information from the study revealed the relevance of a satisfying and active social life in improved overall health. Conversely, it showed and that loneliness in old age adversely affects longevity.

The evidence for links between chronic stress, social isolation, depression and diseases, including cancer, throws a great big monkey wrench into what we thought we knew about maintaining wellness. Just imagine how health advocates need to deal with older adults being more at risk for heart problems and hypertension as a result of social isolation than from diabetes, or how they should address the risks for inflammation being the same in socially isolated teenagers as in kids who don't exercise. The effect of social and psychological factors on the development and progression of disease has been a longstanding hypothesis since ancient times, but the concept that the extent and reach of your social connections can impact your health just as much as diet and exercise is a radical shift from the previously accepted norm.

CHOOSE GRATITUDE

Gratitude has been shown to improve physical and psychological health, increase happiness and reduce depression. It can help diminish negative emotions which when left unchecked can bring on physical toxic stress reactions. People who felt grateful reported experiencing fewer aches and pains than others. They also reported exercising more often and were likely to have regular medical check-ups, which could also contribute to further longevity. No surprises here—being happy should make it easier to be more positive and proactive about your health.

I acknowledge the fact that when life is difficult, gratitude can be difficult. We're not even talking major life challenges here. Sometimes gratitude is just hard to come by. Just pretending to act happy, regardless of what you're feeling, can push your brain to produce positive emotions. If you choose to focus on goodness, you will feel better. Look around for good things. Look everywhere. Smells, colors and sounds can help bring us to a place where we can sense internal gratitude. Once we're feeling it in ourselves, we can begin to spread the love, and express external gratitude. A quote from one of my favorite poets, Mary Oliver, illustrates beautifully how goodness can sometimes lurk in the most unrecognizable of forms: "Someone I loved once gave me a box full of darkness. It took me years to understand that this, too, was a gift."

So when you want to throw cancer some really confusing messages, go celebrate your happiness with friends. Now that you're bathing your cells in green tea antioxidants, maybe cutting back on other dietary and lifestyle vices, getting some exercise, perhaps even finding inner peace in meditation or yoga, the final advantages you can give yourself against cancer are fun and love. Realize gratitude for the present moment and find quality time with your tribe. Just say, "Stand down, cancer. This is my life." And then go steep some tea with your friends.

TEA AS A SOCIAL LUBRICANT

Tea is a great way to get those social connections going. It's a better choice of beverage for a get-together than alcohol, in many ways. You can assert that getting tea-drunk has better social upsides than being mildly inebriated. Tea encourages what one of my favorite tea muses refers to as sparkling conversation. On the flip side, alcohol encourages big, loud talk. Tea helps you focus and remember, whereas with alcohol, our memory tends to go straight out the window. When the most serious stuff hits the fan, I would contend that people prefer to gather intimately around a pot of tea. Alcohol can take the edge off after a rough day at work, but it doesn't comfort in the way that tea does. Theanine is the comfort compound.

The many tea-drinking ceremonies and histories from around the world remind us that tea is much more important as a social beverage than many of us recognize. We might not think of tea as more than something to keep us warm or quench our thirst; in fact, most of us grew up thinking of tea as a weak and drab coffee alternative for grannies. But one-third of the world's population enjoys it as a part of their every day, often as the central beverage to a soothing social occasion. Its many styles of preparation and service are as incredibly fascinating as its many flavors—ranging from the profoundly spiritual Japanese tea ceremony to a barter or business negotiation in Marrakech.

TEA FOR ROMANCE

There are many aromatic, edible, stimulating, relaxing and hallucinogenic substances named after Aphrodite, the Greek goddess of love, used in the belief that they increase sexual desire. The oil of bergamot in Earl Grey, it turns out, has long been used as an aromatic aphrodisiac to reduce muscle tension, anxiety and stress. For added smoothness, add a touch of licorice root, considered an excellent edible and aromatic aphrodisiac. In fact, traditional Chinese medicine used licorice root to enhance love and lust and the ancient Kama Sutra included it as an ingredient for many recipes to increase sexual vigor. According to research done at the Smell and Taste Treatment and Research Foundation in Chicago, the smell of licorice root is particularly stimulating to women.

The visual beauty of rosebuds, coupled with their strong aromatic quality, have often been used as a calming tea, as well as ingredients in calming bath oils, candles and fragrances. But research unveils that rosebuds may do more than simply calm us down. Rosebuds are, indeed, an aphrodisiac. Their aroma stimulates the brain and keeps the mind focused and alert. They're also a great mood enhancer and amplify the libido. Rose essence is said to increase blood flow through the body and fosters a sense of warm stimulation. Jasmine is also an aromatic aphrodisiac.

Needless to say, the caffeine in tea can offer an energy boost at the end of a long day to get you back to your best when starting your evening with your sweetheart. As busy and hectic as modern lifestyles are, we don't always have the time or energy for a leisurely 6 o'clock drink. And sometimes you could use a little bit of a lift heading into the evening. You should consider a romantic tea break next time you come home. A great way to reconnect with your partner at the end of the day is over an aromatic pot of Earl Grey or green jasmine tea.

Just keep in mind the quote by the travel writer Catherine Donzel: "Each cup of tea represents an imaginary voyage." Put out a small vase of flowers in varied colors exuding delicious fragrance, or a candle. They'll share their perfume with the tea as it steeps and contribute to the lovely feeling of romance in the air.

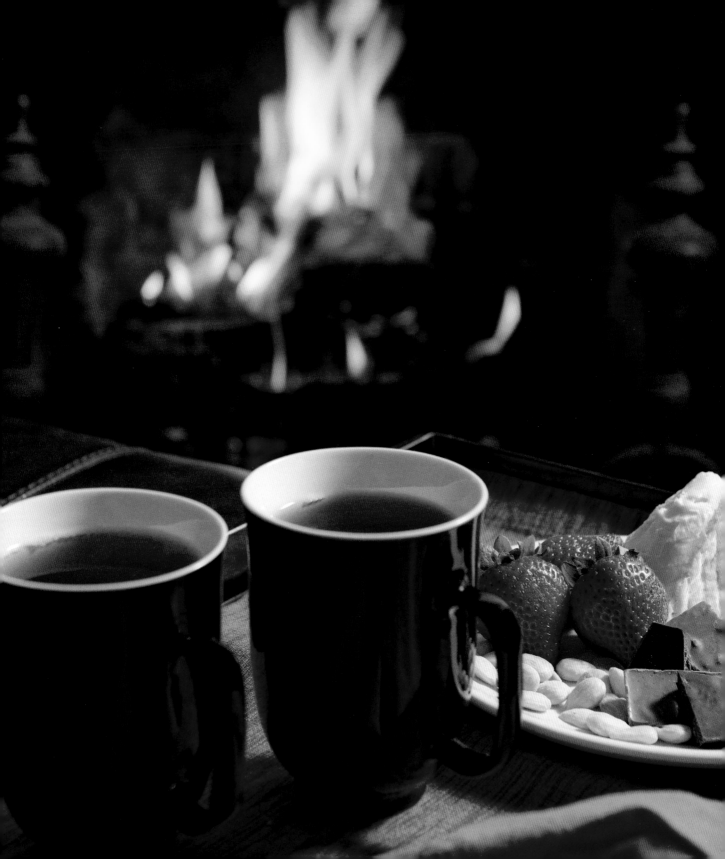

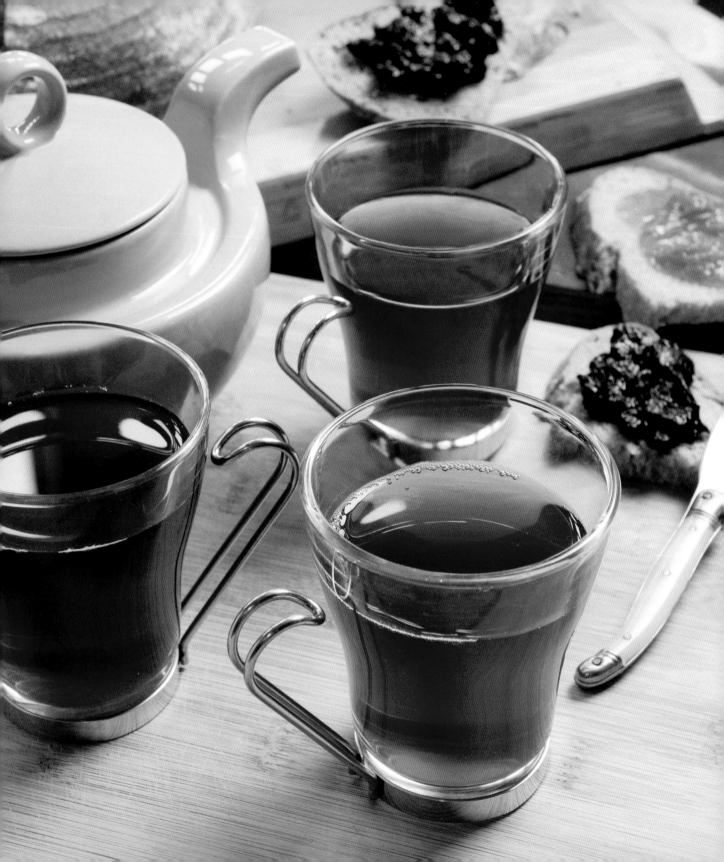

FOUR EASY WAYS TO HAVE A TEA PARTY WITH FRIENDS

Afternoon Tea You don't have to be an Escoffier-trained chef to pull off a tea party that will delight and wow your companions. The secret's in the tea! Your friends will be so dazzled by drinking real tea that they won't obsess over the food. Just put out some breadsticks and cheeses, along with some cut fruit and veggies. Even some fancy little finger sandwiches aren't a huge chore to prepare ahead of time. You can make it a garden tea by taking the show outdoors and adding some herbs or flowers as a centerpiece to your steeped pot of aromatic tea. For truly special occasions, open your tea party with a glass of champagne.

Tea Tasting Party If you're really not into the food prep, take it up a step with your tea and get your guests buzzing with a selection of fresh-brewed teas. If you steep up three exquisite pots of tea, you barely need any snacks at all. Some pumpkin seeds, nuts and dried fruit and any other finger foods are all you need. Put out little cups, and have your friends sip and compare teas of different types and flavors, maybe from different countries. It's like bringing an exotic adventure into your own home, and will definitely fuel some questions and conversation.

Go to a Teahouse Make your tea party an outing. Teahouses tend to be tranquil yin energy places where you can relax, take a deep breath and really connect with your tea and your friends. By contrast, coffee bars are where yang energy tends to be dominant, with lots of people focused on their work, their computers and getting themselves wired.

Party like it's the 21st Century If many of your friends and family live far away, then what about throwing a video chat party? Have one or more people choose their favorite tea and join you to steep, sip and connect. It's even fun to watch what teapots and cups they're using to get it ready. If you've been geeking out with your tea ceremonies, you can show off your newly honed skills. Maybe you'll even get someone else hooked!

AFTER-SCHOOL TEA WITH KIDS — A DRINK WITH JAM AND BREAD

Not only is afternoon tea with your kids a benefit to you, it's also a great way to begin establishing some great social and health habits in your family. For me, this came about not by design or through some great foresight, but because for a while it was the only window of time in the day that I could consistently gear up for and be at my best. Everyone who's had the experience of cancer surgery and chemotherapy knows about the long, long road back to finding your energy, not to mention your taste buds, your body and your hair! But during this process, you don't stop being a mother, and you don't stop wanting to be an asset to your family. Time still flows, consistently, no matter what kind of a compromised schedule you might be on. It was so vitally important for me to keep doing whatever I could to see that my daughters were safe, happy and thriving. When I was working on a limited reserve of energy during my recovery, I would often fall asleep right after dinner, and sometimes even the dinner hour was a bit of a disaster. The only time of day that I could ensure I was up for was right after school, which we made our tea time. The daily tradition became a hearty after-school snack, generally tea with jam and bread, and most importantly, wonderful conversation. We each took turns in describing our highlights and challenges of the day. What I noticed was that since our tea times were right after the school day, all the joys and pains were still fresh, and I got a better insight into their days than if the conversations had taken place later in the evening. The tea selection was a collective decision, as was the choice of teapot. Deciding what to steep and how to serve it was part of this daily celebration. Those choices had a lot to do with the bread or toppings we'd be eating, and got my daughters thinking about food pairings, textures and flavors at an early age.

Bread features prominently in almost all cultures across the world, as does tea. So naturally they go together in metaphor as well as in spirit. Tea with bread makes a delectable feast with just the right cup and a simple slice of the right stuff. As the late James Beard said, "Good bread is the most fundamentally satisfying of all foods; and good bread with fresh butter, the greatest of all feasts." (We tea lovers would contend, with the right cuppa!) Some foods taste better with some breads, and the same rings true for tea and breads. Artisan breads can make a modern tea-time party a snap when paired with the right tea and served up with some butter or jam. Unlike uniform, rectangular breads with soft crumb and crust, artisan breads can contain whole grains, fresh herbs, fruits, nuts and honey. With the wide range of breads and loose-leaf teas available to us today, the variations and combinations are remarkable. What are the main characteristics we're aware of when we taste a new bread? Flavor, of course, but grain and texture are also key. I found these two elements to play more strongly with various tea types than one might guess. In particular, one of the most subtle aspects of a tea's profile, the mouth-coat, is significant when looking at the finer points of a tea-and-bread pairing. Some of our favorites are below:

Classic French Baguette Go classic on the tea side with a nice long-leaf Ceylon black tea. The tea's tannic overtones pair well with the crunchy crust.

Sourdough Great with Assam! The sweetly dry flavor and honey-like mouth-coat in the tea make it pair superbly well with the tangy bite of the bread. Try it also with smoky black teas such as lapsang souchong, Russian caravan or a smoky green gunpowder tea.

Ciabatta, Foccacia Sencha green tea is beautiful here, especially if you're serving it with goat cheese, topped with a touch of matcha and sea salt.

Challah Love this bread with Keemun. Both tea and bread are really round and happy together on the palate.

Unleavened breads (chapatti, roti, pita) Perhaps this is a cultural choice, or maybe that's what makes it work, but these breads pair very well with black teas from Assam and Yunnan, and Moroccan mint green tea.

Honey Wheat Pairs oh so smoothly and beautifully with a black Nilgiri or Ceylon tea, as well as Earl Grey. A nice green tea here is dragonwell, or a green Earl Grey.

Pumpernickel Rye Finds its match with a smoky breakfast blend such as Russian caravan or green gunpowder.

Walnut This bread needs a flavored, non-smoky black. Earl Grey or blackberry tea are both heavenly here.

Pretzel (bread) Lovely with pu-erh tea.

Grisini (bread sticks) Also a natural with pu-erh! And if you're going caffeine-free, they're great with rooibos.

A note about children and caffeine: Caffeine intake in kids has skyrocketed (up 70 percent over the past 30 years) since the advent of sodas, and more recently, energy drinks. Two-thirds of all American children consume caffeine daily, at an average of over 100 mg daily. And sadly, most of the caffeinated beverages kids drink are nutritionally empty calories, loaded with sugar. This is a growing health issue. Caffeine in kids can trigger insomnia and bring on physical fatigue, by boosting the perception of "increased energy." There's no suggested safe level of caffeine for kids. The American Academy of Pediatrics has stated that caffeinated energy drinks should be eliminated from children's diets. Caffeine consumption approaching 1,000 mg in kids has caused hospitalization and been believed to bring on cardiac arrhythmia. Health Canada's recommendation for children under 12 is no more than 2.5 mg of caffeine for every kilogram of body weight. That would amount to about 50 mg of caffeine for a 5-year-old child. For larger adolescents, 150 to 250 mg of caffeine daily is likely safe medically. One 8-ounce (240-ml) cup of green tea or a 12-ounce (355-ml) can of cola each contain about 35 mg caffeine. A cup of black tea has 40 to 45 mg caffeine. Milk tea, made with half milk, half tea would cut that amount in two; and a kid's-size cup would take it down proportionally even more. Also, there are many wonderful herbal tisanes that are caffeine-free.

Throw a Stress-Free Holiday Tea Party

If it's that time of year, you can throw a traditional holiday sweets tea party. You can go as fancy as you like, but there are easy ways to get festive with a tea party as well. Serve up at least two different types of tea. It's always good to have a caffeine-free variety, and peppermint is a great holiday choice. Then steep up a pot of your own favorite tea. The best part of holiday entertaining isn't gifting, but sharing, and tea lovers do like to share their latest tea finds. Serving suggestions follow:

Milk chocolate and truffles pair supremely well with Darjeeling, as a contrast in textures. The sweet, smooth and buttery chocolate (imagine ganache) juxtaposed with the bright and lightly earthy tea flavor enhances the milk chocolate and brings it to a higher level of sophistication.

Dark chocolate pairs supremely well with green and white teas. It's like a point-counterpoint theme at work here to help you pick up on subtle notes in the chocolates. Some dark chocolates have strong citrus notes. Nothing tops a citrus-scented green tea here. For the smoothest of super dark chocolates (more than 70% cacao) a fantastic pairing is white tea, or a white tea blend.

Peanut brittle resonates brilliantly with the brisk, ocean-like flavor of a fresh green sencha tea.

Caramel works in your mouth like the smoothest of chocolates. Try this with a white tea blend or a single-estate white tea. It's like heaven on clouds . . .

Pumpkin pie can be paired with either a spice tea or an unflavored black tea. It also works well with pure or spiced caffeine-free rooibos.

Pecan pie's hands-down favorite would be Darjeeling. It's also great with any tea with vanilla or almond.

And as you're looking for the right tea to serve with an assortment of cookies or rugelach, you need look no further than to Earl Grey. It is the prince among princes at your holiday tea parties. The subtle citrus-bergamot helps the various flavors, spices, fruits and nuts come to life.

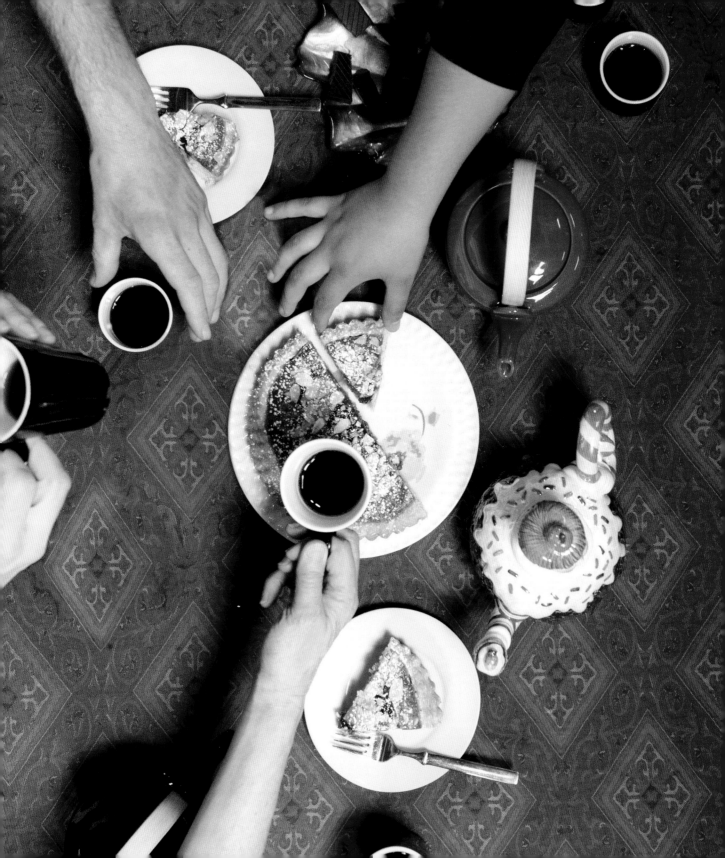

-PART FOUR-

LET'S TELL CANCER OFF NOW!

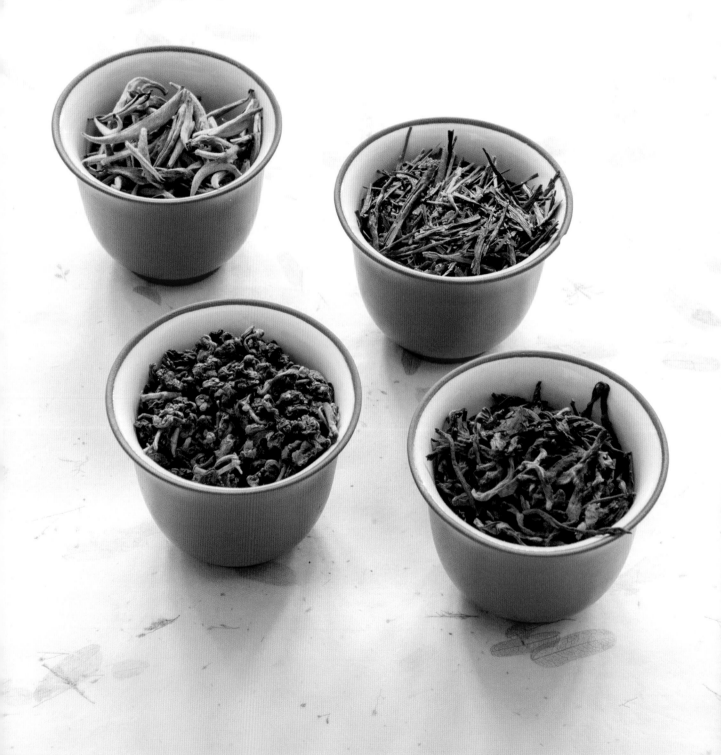

Chapter 9

IT'S YOUR TEA TIME

YOUR EVERY DAY IS THE MOST IMPORTANT DAY

Buzz off, cancer. Your deranged cells have no place in my body. From now on, we play on my terms, and you've got another thing coming if you think I'm going to make myself an easy target!

So now that we've learned the basics of how to live a life that shuns cancer, let's get right down to learning how to make tea easy, accessible and fun and how to make this daily immunity-boosting tea habit your reality. In this chapter you'll find all the practical how-to info to guide you through.

If you don't get in all the tea servings you'd hoped for on some days, don't stress about it! One cup of tea a day is already better than none. Any fresh, whole leaf tea you're bringing into your day is a major step in a positive direction. If you stick with the program, even semi-consistently, tea will become a new presence in your life and before you know it, that 5-cup-a-day habit will just establish itself without too much counting needed on your part.

Before you start, get ready! Set up your tea pantry. Go shopping for some whole leaf teas either in a tea shop or online. Developing a relationship with a tea merchant who knows their stuff can be super helpful and open your horizons to teas you would otherwise have never stumbled upon.

DRINK LIKE A RUSSIAN

We know that the Chinese love to drink tea, and so do the Irish and the Brits. But Russians are known for drinking vodka, right? Actually, Russians drink more tea per capita than people in either China or Japan. The Russians have become such devoted tea drinkers that as a nation they are among the largest consumers of tea in the world. Favorite Russian-style tea blends are sometimes slightly smoked, or flavored with citrus fruits and bergamot, and include romantic names such as Russian Caravan and Czar Alexander. As a first generation American and daughter of Russian immigrants, I grew up steeped in Russian tea traditions. And I can't imagine a Russian home without the samovar, even if just as a relic on display from the family's history. The samovar is a combination of a bubbling hot water heater and a teapot. Literally meaning self-cooker, it's a simple, but highly effective, piece of equipment that makes warm tea available throughout the day. It functions by heating a metal urn of water through a central tube heated by a charcoal or wood fire.

The samovar is lovingly referred to in Russian literary works and often appears in paintings and historical photographs. You can't get through any Tolstoy story without mention of one: "In the summer, the samovar would sit on a table in the garden; in winter, it might be brought inside, with a long pipe for the smoke to escape directly into the chimney of the house." A strong concentrate of tea (*zavarka*) sits on top of the metal urn, staying warm and is diluted bit by bit throughout the day, as needed, each time tea is served. The samovar was a purely Russian invention, although its design is based on that of Mongolian kettles. I have very few remaining things that my family brought with them when they escaped from Russia during World War II, but the heaviest and clunkiest of these is a big, heavy metal samovar. I can't imagine why they chose to haul something such as that along—when carrying everything you own on yourself—but they did, and here it sits now, in our conference room at work. Probably not an evening went by, wherever they were on that journey, without the samovar bubbling, and had tea with something sweet on the side, either a cube of sugar, candied fruit or a spoonful of preserves.

Vipyem chayu? (Shall we have tea?)

DETERMINE YOUR TEA TYPE

The more you discover about what makes your taste buds happy, the more you'll take enjoyment in your daily tea ritual. In Part One of this book we touched on the different tea types and how they're made with different processes and varying levels of oxidation (page 27). The versatility of the tea leaf offers almost endless possibilities for your cuppa, but in the end, what you steep and how you steep it will come down to your personal preference. Experiment a bit to find out what you like. You might decide that you like your black tea extra bold, but your green tea more on the light side. You might also find that you dream about those sweet, smooth Chinese green teas, but turn your nose up at the lively, grassy Japanese greens. Adding herbals, fruits and florals to your teas opens up more flavor twists and combinations.

And what to do if after you've tried a few different tea types you're really not digging the taste of the teas you've tried thus far? Try stepping back a bit and easing your way into it by cutting the tea with other ingredients, either in the form of a tea latte, or mixed with other beverages. You can even extend your reach to new tea types using this trick.

If you start with a traditional Arnold Palmer (one part lemonade, one part iced tea) with the usual Ceylon black tea, try transitioning the tea part after a while, say with either green jasmine or dragonwell that will connect you more deeply to the green tea flavors.

If you can't decide where to start, see if either of these selection guides can help steer you to some options that sound good—because really, it's all about you.

A QUIZ TO HELP PICK YOUR TEA

Choose the most appealing answer to help guide you in your tea choice:

1. Snack time, and you get to choose from five plates of fruits:
a. Apples and Pears
b. Peaches and Apricots
c. Strawberries and Mangoes
d. Blackberries, Plums and Raisins
e. Melons and Cherries

2. It's time for dinner, and you're hungry:
a. Grilled cheese or grilled chicken
b. Quiche, or salmon with salad
c. Grilled veggies or sushi
d. Pasta with marinara sauce, or steak and potatoes
e. Spicy Indian, Mexican or Asian

3. Pick one of these salad dressings from the menu:
a. Ranch
b. Honey Mustard
c. Vinaigrette
d. Blue Cheese
e. Raspberry

4. For wine lovers only:
a. Pinot Grigio or Sauvignon Blanc
b. Chardonnay, Late Harvest Riesling
c. Merlot, Pinot Noir, Chianti, Rioja, Valpolicella, Beaujolais
d. Cabernet Sauvignon, Nebbiolo, Barolo, Barbaresco, Malbec
e. Burgundy, Rose

(continued)

A QUIZ TO HELP PICK YOUR TEA (CONTINUED)

5. Cheers to the beers:

a. American-style Pilsners, such as Coors, Bud or Rolling Rock

b. Hefeweizens, Witbiers or Belgians

c. Pale Ales or bitter IPAs

d. Porters or Stouts

e. Sour beers

6. Choose the flavor profile that makes your mouth water:

a. Fruit-forward, floral, smooth, clean

b. Ripe fruit, honey, buttery, roasted

c. Seaweed, umami, sweetly grassy, citrus

d. Earthy, cocoa, smoky, malty, peppery

e. Woody, sweet, spicy, vanilla

7. Your dream dessert would be:

a. Apple Pie or Lemon Meringue Pie

b. Creme Brûlée, Vanilla or Coconut Ice Cream

c. Chocolate mousse or Chocolate Chip Cookies

d. Pumpkin or Pecan Pie, Flourless Chocolate Cake

e. Berry Sorbet or a Tart Fruit Pie

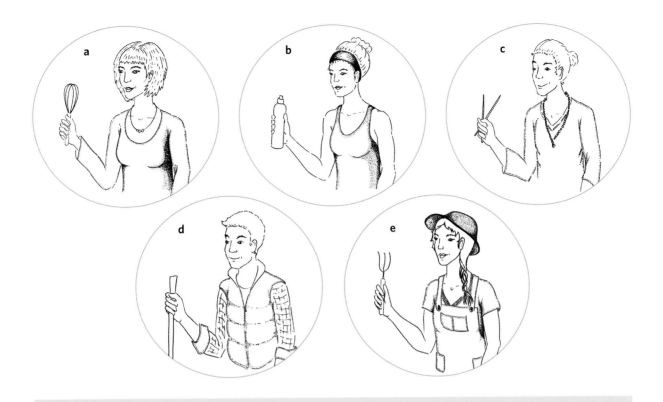

ANSWERS

Mostly a's? If you're into book clubs, dancing and baking, and your ideal vacation is on a yacht, vacationing in the Bahamas or the British Virgin Islands, try flavored and floral green teas such as jasmine and citrus, or Keemun, English breakfast and Earl Grey black teas.

Mostly b's? If you're into long walks, yoga and wine tastings, and your ideal leisure time would be a gourmet picnic in the countryside, try Chinese green and white teas, or oolong teas—such as dragonwell, clouds and mist, white peony, white silver needles and Iron Goddess of Mercy (Ti Kwan Yin) oolong tea.

Mostly c's? If you're into dinner parties, meditation and sushi, and your ideal getaway would be scuba diving in beautiful, exotic places, try Japanese green teas such as sencha, bancha, gyokuro and matcha or Darjeeling and Ceylon black teas.

Mostly d's? If you're into happy hour, hiking and BBQing, and your ideal adventure would be a high-altitude trek, try strong black teas such as Assam, Yunnan, lapsang souchong, Irish breakfast or pu-erh; and gunpowder, genmaicha or hojicha green teas.

Mostly e's? If you're into crafting, gardening and game night, and your ideal evening would be a romantic evening in front of a cozy fireplace, try flavored and/or spicy black teas such as chocolate cherry, ginger peach, cinnamon spice or chai. If you're in the mood for a plain, classic tea, go for a Nilgiri black tea.

Another way you can select your teas is by tea type and caffeine content. If you're weaning yourself off coffee to get your tea in, you may want to find some of the more highly caffeinated teas, such as pu-erhs and black teas to best fill in for the cup of joe you're foregoing. On the other hand, if you're sensitive to caffeine, and struggling with trying to figure out how to get five servings of tea in your day without spiraling out of control, you can do that with relative ease if you stick to white and green teas. A combination of five 8-ounce (240-ml) servings of those teas shouldn't exceed that of a single serving of coffee. And if you really can't tolerate caffeine at all, just stick to cold brewing green and white teas. Five cups (1.2 L) of those in cold brews will likely yield less than half the caffeine of a single cup of coffee.

Type	Flavor Profiles	Caffeine/Serving	Caffeine compared to 1 cup of coffee
White	Subtle, slightly sweet, floral or vegetal	10–15 mg	$\frac{1}{10}$
Green	Lively, vegetal, toasty or grassy	20–30 mg	$\frac{1}{5}$
Matcha	Thick, slightly sweet, umami	25–35 mg	$\frac{1}{4}$
Oolong	Complex, sweet, floral or toasty	20–40 mg	$\frac{1}{5}$–$\frac{1}{4}$
Black	Full-bodied, fruity, honey, malty or roasty, spicy or cocoa	40–50 mg	$\frac{1}{3}$
Pu-erh	Very full mouth-coat, fruity, woody, caramel	50–70 mg	$\frac{1}{2}$

HOW TO GET THE BEST BREW FROM THAT BADASS *CAMELLIA SINENSIS*

Perhaps the most daunting part of getting into loose leaf tea is the need for something beyond a cup and a tea bag. First step: Chillax. This isn't new—people have been steeping tea for almost 5,000 years, and billions of people steep real tea leaves without fancy accessories every day.

What you'll need:

1. Tea leaves

2. Water, hot or cold, depending on which steeping method you choose

3. Heat-resistant vessel to steep in such as a mug, teapot or a mason jar

4. Filter or strainer to separate the leaves from your drink when done steeping

What to do:

1. Place tea leaves in your steeping vessel

2. Get water to the right temp for your tea

3. Pour water over leaves to steep

4. Strain the leaves out

HOT BREW STEEPING GUIDE

This is a guide that works well as a first-time steep. But if you don't like your tea the first time you make it, try steeping it with a bit more tea leaves and a little cooler water, and/or for a little less time.

Tea Type	Leaves per 8 oz (240 ml) Water	Water Temp	Steep Time
White	1 heaping tsp (2.5 g)	175°F (80°C) (or boil, pour, wait 3 minutes)	2 to 3 minutes*
Green	1 rounded tsp (2.3 g)	175°F (80°C) (or boil, pour, wait 3 minutes)	2 to 3 minutes*
Oolong	1 rounded tsp (2.3 g)	195°F (90°C) (or boil, pour, wait 3 minutes)	2 to 3 minutes*
Black	1 tsp (2 g)	boiling	3 to 5 minutes
Pu-erh	1 tsp (2 g)	boiling	2 to 5 minutes*

*Multiple steeps—For many teas, you can re-infuse the same leaves two or more times. Just leave them to steep about a minute longer with each subsequent infusion.

PERFECT TEA WITHOUT A DIGITAL KETTLE

In the above chart are some guidelines for getting your water to the right temperature simply by boiling the water and letting it cool down a bit. There's another way to get there without a thermometer: an ancient Chinese method which is a great trick to know and works remarkably well. There are three key temperature ranges for steeping teas: 175°F (80°C) for white and green teas, 195°F (90°C) for oolong teas and boiling for black and pu-erh teas. The saying goes "a watched pot never boils," but did you know that you can actually see water get to those temps? Pour your freshly drawn water into a pot, and heat it on the stove. Just don't get distracted and wander off!

As soon as you see individual "fish eyes" at the bottom of the pot, your water's at the right temperature for white teas. Pairs of them appearing means go for green. Those fish eyes are nucleation sites appearing in the process of boiling. Translation: That's water changing states and the resulting vapor bubbles overcoming the heavier weight of liquid water.

When you see "strings of pearls" beginning to rise up from those nucleation sites (you'll know exactly what they are when you see them) your water's ready to steep oolong teas. This is honestly one of my favorite things about making darjeeling.

"Raging river" is the visual cue for boiling point—your water is experiencing a phase change full on ba-da-boom! This is the turbulence your black teas and pu-erh need to infuse their tough, oxidized leaves.

JUST FORGET THE HOT WATER AND COLD BREW IT!

If you're still totally put off by the need for precision and using a measuring spoon and timer, you might be one of us who is better suited for brewing your teas cold. That's not a bad thing! Cold brewing a fine loose leaf tea is easier than hot brewing it and results in a sublime and equally healthy brew.

So how do you cold brew? Nothing could be simpler. You can cold brew whole leaf tea in the fridge using cold water and a pitcher, mason jar or water bottle. You can even cold brew fresh tea on-the-go. Because cold brewing is a more forgiving process, proportions and steeping times aren't as critical as when you're hot brewing. Cold brewing always produces a well-balanced tea without bitterness or clouding. When you use cool water, the leaves infuse more slowly and you don't run the risk of overstepping your tea. The good news: Your polyphenol molecules infuse just as happily in cold water, as they do in hot, albeit more slowly.

One point about fresh, cold-brewed tea, however, is that it is just that—FRESH. With no citric acid or preservatives added, it's not something that you should leave to drink days later. Drink your cold brew within 24 hours, and don't leave your cold brew sitting out in the sun. Cold brewing—either in the refrigerator or at room temperature without added heat—is safe for any tea type because the final heated phase in tea processing introduces a natural enzyme "kill" step to inhibit further bacterial growth in the leaf.

COLD BREW STEEPING GUIDE

1. Add 2 heaping tablespoons (10 g) loose leaf tea to 32 ounces (960 ml) fresh cold water in pitcher or mason jar

2. Steep for 30 minutes to 1 hour in the fridge, or for 10 to 30 minutes at room temperature

3. Strain the leaves out and serve straight or over ice

Note: If you have a bottle with a tea filter, you can serve or drink your cold brew straight from the bottle without straining out the leaves.

White teas steep like they were made to be cold brewed. These are the teas that have been shown to yield even higher antioxidant properties when cold brewed versus hot.

Green teas are absolutely exquisite when cold brewed. This is where many green teas really shine their sweeter side. The same teas that require the utmost precision in temperature and timing to not go bitter when brewed hot are usually a breeze to cold brew. And for my money, it's the best aspects of their flavor which are most prominent in their cold water extractions.

Oolong teas only need the slightest amount of tea leaves to go a very long way in a cold brew.

Black teas don't cold brew easily. Their leaves are tough and need hot water in order to extract well. Black tea leaves don't re-steep well either, as most of their flavor comes out in that first soak in boiling water. If you want to cold brew a black tea, plan on leaving it to brew overnight, otherwise it will be very light. Many people actually prefer the flavor of black teas cold brewed, as they come out much sweeter with less tannin.

Pu-erh teas, by contrast to black teas, cold brew nicely. They'll taste absolutely fabulous either black or with a small splash of creamer, ice latte style.

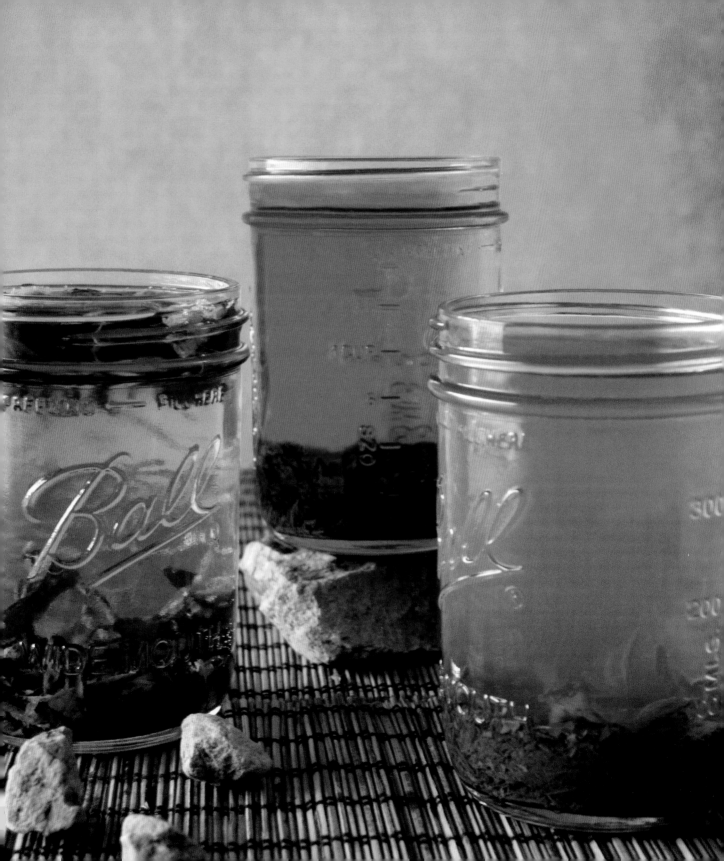

THE BEGINNER'S TEA PANTRY

Now that you're familiar with the guidelines for how to steep any tea every possible way, what do you really need to have on hand to get your healthy brew going? You'd be surprised how little you need beyond tea and water—there are just a few basic things, most of which are probably already within your reach, which you'll need in order to make that epic cup of tea and sip in style. Chances are, you won't need to spend a dime beyond what your purchase of tea leaves will cost.

1. Decent Leaves Make sure you have fresh, quality tea on hand. Remember: Your tea should look like it came from a plant, not a dustpan. You can mess up a great tea, but you probably won't ever make a mediocre tea taste phenomenal. Go chase down some quality *Camellia sinensis*.

2. Good Water A great cup of tea requires pure water. Remember that it makes up over 99 percent of your beverage, so water quality is as critical as that of the tea leaves. Start with fresh, preferably filtered water. Ideally, you could get nicely oxygenated water straight out of the faucet. If you don't have a water filter, or don't like your tap water, you can use bottled water. Don't use distilled water, though; it's been so depleted that it'll make your tea taste perfectly flat.

3. Temperature and Perfect Timing You'd be surprised how quickly a really great tea can begin to taste like overcooked Brussels sprouts when steeped too hot or too long. Use a timer. Luckily most kitchens come equipped with timers on the microwave or stove, so the heavy thinking can be left to them. I'll be honest: Sometimes (often), I unintentionally over-steep my tea until it tastes bitter. It can often be salvaged by adding a bit more water to the brew to thin it out a bit. A digital kettle makes getting the right water temp brainless, but you can also go the ancient Chinese route of actually watching your water come to the right temperature, or use the boil and wait a few minutes method.

4. **Steeping Vessel** I love ceramic because it holds heat well and because it doesn't impart any flavor on the tea. Glass is great too, but it's not as effective for heat retention. For cold brewing, when heat doesn't matter of course, I almost always brew tea in mason jars or a glass cold brew bottle. Some teas can get a funny flavor from certain metals, which can leave a strange taste in your tumbler especially when you're brewing your tea right in it. That said, many of the newer double-walled stainless steel tumblers are great for keeping tea either hot or cold for hours. Watch out, though, it's just not fun to sip from hot metal so be careful if you're making your tea in a stainless tumbler. With time, you'll figure out your favorite tea steepers. I own a bunch, and always come back to my favorite few.

5. Strainer or Infuser You don't need to go high tech here. Most people making tea around the world don't use any fancy contraptions to separate the tea leaves from the water when they're done steeping. There are plenty of times when I've made tea, either at a friend's house or while on travel, with the water heated in a plain old pot, steeped in another pot and then strained out using the lid into cups. Any old clean strainer will work great too. An infuser is the other way to go. You put your tea leaves in and remove it after you're finished steeping your tea. You've likely seen the tea-balls on chains that look like a Christmas ornament with holes, but there are hundreds of products out there for steeping tea. The tea balls work just fine for a cup of tea, but it's preferable to have a steeper with a larger volume to allow water to flow more freely between the leaves. The extra volume allows the tea leaves to completely unfurl, releasing their full flavor, aroma and goodness.

6. Tea Storage Tea stays fresh for longer if it is properly stored in a sealed, light-proof container, such as a tea tin or an air-tight canister. Keep it stashed away from heat, light, humidity or extreme cold.

HOW TO GET YOUR IMMUNITY-BOOSTING TEA GAME ON

You might be thinking, when the heck am I supposed to find the time to make and drink five servings of tea? It all works better if you keep it as easy as possible on yourself. Sure, your health is Job #1, but we don't need this new tea leaf steeping fiasco to consume your whole damn day, do we? Five cups of tea a day may seem like you're taking on a second career at first, but with the right tools and info, you can make it ridiculously simple. Here are some tricks on how to get your body's share of ass-kicking, calm-seeking, fitness-loving tea into your every day.

Your first cup in the morning: You don't need to ditch the pot of coffee, not just yet, at least, although a cup of tea will do just as well to energize you for the day without your mid-morning caffeine crash. For now, just try a cup of your favorite black or green tea before your cup of coffee to get your engines running.

On the road: If you're like most Americans, you spend too much time in the car getting to and from work. Bringing tea on your commute is a great opportunity to lay off the horn and turn your road rage into a mini meditation.

Take a tea break from your computer: Don't just give your eyes a well-needed break, refresh your mind and refill on antioxidants at the same time with a tea break. You'll be surprised at how much a cup of green tea and a walk can clear your head. And if you really can't afford to break away today, steep and re-steep your favorite white, green or oolong tea at your desk. It will make it feel like you're taking a break!

Say "Hasta Mañana" to the workday: Tea is the perfect way to unwind and reboot before getting into your evening. If you're not out indulging in a glass of wine for happy hour with friends, steep yourself a favorite tea to celebrate the end of the work day.

Add tea to your exercise routine: Supercharge your workouts with an energy and a metabolic boost. Enjoy some tea thirty minutes before you start any physical activity. Then help restore your muscles and your soul with tea post-workout.

You want to refresh that tea polyphenol level in your bloodstream every few hours, so it's good to start first thing in the morning, then keep coming back to refuel that supply throughout the day. Don't obsess about pairing it with your meals; remember that tea is best absorbed on an empty stomach.

GET TEA FIT IN 3 WEEKS

This plan, streamlined for real life, will ease you into a full-on tea habit. Within three weeks, your body should start to feel and show the benefits from the tea that is now working in your system 24/7. You will feel amazing. The series of little sips will indulge your senses with new flavor sensations while simultaneously nurturing your wellness. The power of habit is strong. Just keep steeping according to plan for three weeks, and by the time you're through, tea will have become a welcome part of your every day. PS: The fun part—the choice of which teas to steep—is left entirely up to you!

WEEK ONE: 3 SERVINGS PER DAY (1 SERVING = 8 OUNCES [240 ML] = 1 CUP)

Serving 1: Drink 8 ounces (240 ml) Early Morning, Pre-Coffee, Pre-Breakfast

Steep up a fresh cup of tea before you begin your morning routine. This start is the key cup of tea in your day—your cells' phytochemical beverage wake-up call—that's why it's important to have this one before you eat or drink anything else.

Tip: Pu-erh teas have the highest caffeine yield to help get your day going.

Servings 2-3: Sip 16 ounces (480 ml) Throughout Your Day

Water is life. Infuse it with the goodness of the tea leaf. Either enhance a bottle of water with tea by cold brewing or steep up two servings and take it with you, hot or chilled, in a tumbler. If you're sensitive to caffeine, you may want to finish sipping these before 4 PM.

Tip: Roasted green teas are super easy on your stomach and low in caffeine.

WEEK TWO: 4 SERVINGS PER DAY

Serving 1: Drink 8 ounces (240 ml) Early Morning, Pre-Coffee, Pre-Breakfast

Same as Week One

Servings 2-3: Sip 16 ounces (480 ml) Throughout Your Day

Same as Week One

Serving 4: Drink 8 ounces (240 ml) Late Morning, One Hour Before Lunch

Steep up a cup of tea for a late morning tea break. If it's totally impractical for you to get this done during the day, steep up two servings for your early AM tea and either drink it all then, or bring it along for this tea break.

WEEK THREE: 5 SERVINGS PER DAY

Serving 1: Drink 8 ounces (240 ml) Early Morning, Pre-Coffee, Pre-Breakfast

Same as Weeks One & Two

Tip: Try a dessert tea before breakfast.

Servings 2-3: Sip 16 ounces (480 ml) Throughout Your Day

Same as Weeks One & Two

Tip: Bring a little variety to your tea by adding fruits or herbals.

Serving 4: Drink 8 ounces (240 ml) Late Morning, One Hour Before Lunch

Same as Week Two

Tip: If you're looking for a metabolism boost before lunch, steep up a green, white or oolong tea.

Serving 5: Drink 8 ounces (240 ml) Afternoon Break, Pre- or Post-Workout

Add your fifth tea serving either as an afternoon tea break, or as part of an exercise routine. Alternatively, you can choose to increase the amount of the tea you're sipping during the day—just bump that two serving bottle up to three servings.

Check in with your energy and stress levels. You may very well feel less of a pull toward your morning coffee after three weeks of sipping tea throughout the day. Coffee is a legitimate healthy plant-based beverage in its own right, but now that you've boosted your tea intake, you may want to see the effects of cutting back. Many people report sleeping better and having less afternoon fatigue when they're not drinking coffee. If you choose not to give up that morning cup of joe with your new found tea habit, you should keep tabs on your overall caffeine intake and try to keep the coffee to just one cup (240 ml) daily.

REPEAT AFTER ME

Hello, Beautiful! Making it through your first 21 days with tea is a huge leap toward taking control of your own health. You've now proved that things don't have to stay the same. Creating a good habit doesn't take more work than building a bad habit. It's all about repetition. In the case of making a positive change, you're paving a path of caring and understanding of your body, as an investment in better health, longevity and vitality. Once you realize that you really care, which is ironically often prompted by an episode of disease, you can begin to understand and then act. To quote one of my favorite teachers: "If you can, you must."

Steep on.

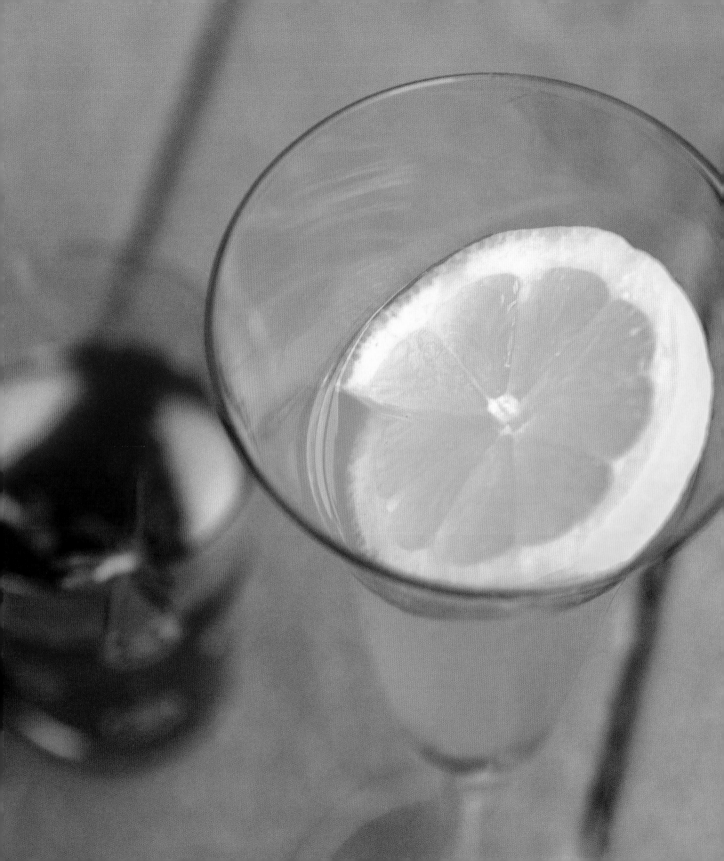

Chapter 10

SIP ON THIS, CANCER

THE EXPERT IN ANYTHING WAS ONCE A BEGINNER

Is your head spinning with tea types, water temperatures, spices and tea gadgets? Take a deep breath, and pat yourself on the back. You already now know more about steeping tea than 95 percent of all Americans. You're a pro. But if you have no fear of becoming a true tea geek, read on for some advanced tea savvy and luscious drink recipes.

Developing a palate for tea is an ongoing process. Your palate can always become better trained, and it will do so with every new tea you encounter. Apart from being able to distinguish types, regions, grades, added flavors and scents, which everyone can learn with time and regular tea tastings, there are no right answers. Remember, it's all about you.

So what do pro tasters do when trying a new tea? They engage their senses on multiple fronts—sight, touch, smell and taste. When we do a sensory tea evaluation, we follow the following four basic steps:

1. *Examine the tea leaves for color, luster, size, breakage and freshness.*

2. *Touch the tea leaves to get a closer examination of freshness, sheen and leaf quality.*

3. *Smell the dry tea leaves. Steep. Watch the leaves. Smell again.*

4. *Taste.*

Some of the more common characteristics used to describe tea flavors and aromas are: sweet, woody, smoky, malty, fruity, floral, chocolate, nutty, toasty, spicy, honey, vegetal and umami. The overall attack and body of a tea can range anywhere from subtle and sophisticated, to well-balanced, to multidimensional, to bold and in charge. For me, the essence of the taste of a tea all comes down to mouthfeel. What's the impression that splash made inside your mouth? Often times, how you perceive the texture and astringency of your tea, its intensity and how it lingers make a stronger impression on you than actual nuances in its flavor. One of the best things about loose leaf tea is that its variety becomes just as pleasing as consistency. The journey you'll take with a tea leaf through multiple infusions is a taste adventure. Each steeping will uncover a new facet of that tea's flavor potential. Cold brewing is yet another way to uncover completely new flavor profiles in loose leaf tea.

WHOLE LEAF TEAS AND PRO STEEPING TIPS

There are volumes of information you can find, with poetic descriptions, on tasting and preparing teas, their growing regions and the various cultures and people who cultivate them. If you really get into tea, you'll want to find some of these. Reading them can sometimes feel like a mini journey to some of tea's many beautiful origins. This section is intended to whet your appetite for seeking out and trying new teas by giving you a closer look at some of the world's favorites. They're listed in order of highest caffeine yield to lowest, to help you choose wisely and sip happy any time of day.

PU-ERH

Pu-erh—If you didn't mind the taste of dirt the last time you ate it after flying off your mountain bike, try this tea. I mean that in the kindest way—no matter how many wonderful teas I taste and drink, pu-erh is my fave. It's still the one that gets me every time. This earthy, aged tea is available in both fully oxidized ripe (*shou*) and unoxidized raw (*sheng*) versions. The more commonly exported style is the fully oxidized dark version, and you'll see it in both loose leaf form, or as large or small tea bricks, which look like packaged Frisbees. Little bits of the brick are chiseled off each time you want to steep. Some aged Pu-erhs can yield an infusion the color of dark brown shoe polish. Don't let that get you down—you might find that you're in for an amazing treat! You can make your pu-erh in any teapot or mug you have, but this tea lends itself to clay teapots superbly well. As you continue using the same clay teapot to infuse your pu-erh day after day, the inside of the teapot will become completely coated with the tea, and the outside of the teapot will become shinier and shinier—the sign of a well-seasoned and well-loved Yixing (YEE-shing) clay teapot.

Tip: It's a good idea to rinse the leaves before you steep, through a strainer, since many pu-erhs are aged. You can also just drain your steeping vessel after 10 to 15 seconds before you make your first infusion.

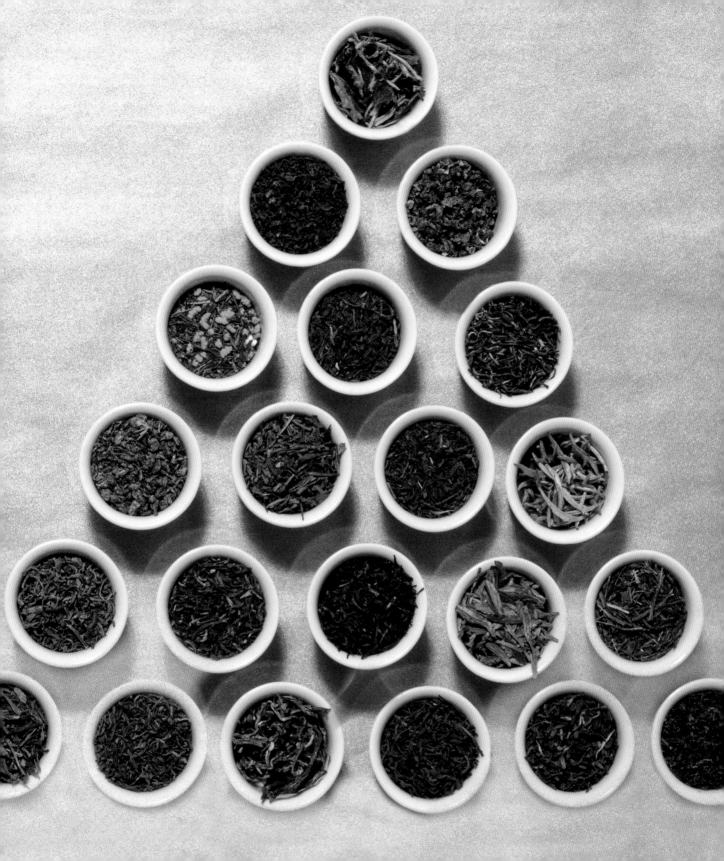

BLACK

Assam Everything about this tea is big, including the plant it grows on and the leaf. The varietal of tea plant indigenous to the Assam region in India is *Camellia sinensis assamica,* which is about twice as big as the Chinese varietal *Camellia sinensis sinensis.* The larger leaves from *assamica* produce a darker and stronger tea, which makes it well suited to milk and sugar. You can always taste the Assam amongst other black teas thanks to its distinctive malty aroma and honey finish. Even though it's a strong tea, Assam can be velvety smooth. Assam is one of only two regions in the world with native tea plants, along with Southern China. This very moist Himalayan valley is over 500 miles (804 km) long, following the Brahmaputra River. Assam gets over 100 inches (3 m) of rainfall annually, and parts of it look like a tropical jungle. It's is also home to the largest wildlife sanctuary in India, where if you're lucky, you can still see the rare, one-horned Indian rhino and the Asiatic elephant.

TIP: If you'd like it stronger, go up in leaf quantity, but don't increase steeping time.

Yunnan Hailing from the southern part of China, Yunnan is powerful and complex. This tea is at the same time spicy-peppery and smooth like chocolate mocha. You might say it's malty rough on the outside and syrupy sweet on the inside. Its twisted, wiry leaves are almost chestnut in color, often with golden yellow tips. Yunnan teas steep up dark, but with a distinctive golden-reddish tint. Heavy in rainfall and humid, this beautiful region that is ideal for growing tea is also one of China's most sought-after clean-air outdoor recreation areas. Yunnan means "South of the Clouds." It's a huge and diverse province, bordering Tibet on the north, and Laos and Vietnam beyond its mountain range to the south.

TIP: Start with your leaf quantity at 1 teaspoon (2 g) per 8 ounces (240 ml) water, and work your way up from there, if needed.

Lapsang Souchong This tea is not for the faint of heart (or palate, for that matter!) but if you just love hanging out by the campfire, it might be love at first sip. People either love it or hate it. (I happen to love it, on occasion!) Lapsang smells and tastes like pure smoke, in a most astounding way—people a block away will be well aware of your cup of lapsang brewing. It's crazy how these little black tea leaves can have so pervasive and powerful an aroma. As a part of their processing, lapsang leaves become thoroughly scented with smoking pinewood. The flavors you can perceive behind the campfire are sweet, fruity and sometimes slightly spicy. Lapsang souchong is cultivated in the Wuyi mountains of Fujian Province, China.

TIP: You're in for an adventure, so just keep an open mind! If you're taken aback, try adding a little splash of maple syrup.

English and Irish Breakfast Blends Tea blends are a path to creating a consistent flavor profile year after year. As individual crops will differ with each season's harvest, using a combination of these teas creates an ensemble tea profile which is easier to replicate. Breakfast blends are the most popular of all tea blends, and most of these use Assam tea to create a warm, smooth and malty base, although many are now incorporating black teas from Kenya as well.

Tip: These teas are blended to offer a strong morning wake-up call to the palate. They will stand up well to milk, if that's how you prefer to take your morning cuppa.

Earl Grey Flavored teas are often thought of as a great gateway to the pure single estate teas. Having something with nice added flavors and aromas can make the taste of tea more accessible to ease into. Earl Grey is the most common flavored tea in the Western world. Its distinctive flavor and fragrance come from oil of bergamot, a Mediterranean citrus fruit, and the black tea base is a blend of teas, which traditionally hail from China, India and/or Sri Lanka. Today, you can find Earl Grey teas on green, white and even oolong tea bases. The origin of the tea's name is presumed to come from Charles Grey, the 2nd Earl Grey, who as the British prime minister in the 1830s was conferred a gift of this exquisite bergamot-scented tea at the conclusion of his diplomatic visit to China.

TIP: Absolutely terrific in a tea latte.

Keemun Keemun is pleasantly rich and balanced without being overpowering. It has an intriguing natural sweetness, with just slight notes of fruit or floral and an aroma reminiscent of toast, maybe even with a tiny smudge of melted chocolate. This distinctive tea is jet black in color, and its classic, superbly balanced body simply sings with flavor and aroma. Keemun is unique in that it's the only tea with myrcenal, a naturally occurring essential oil. Myrcenal is found only in the cultivar of tea plant from which Keemun tea is produced, in Anhui Province, which is known for its many extraordinary green and oolong teas. It's classified as one of China's ten most famous teas. Keemun is like the darling Darjeeling of China, the perfectly balanced ballerina of black teas.

TIP: Enjoy! There's not a lot that can go wrong in steeping Keemun.

Nilgiri The teas from this Southernmost misty, lush and mountainous region of India are among the most approachable of all black teas. They've earned their reputation because they stay crystal clear and don't cloud when chilled, like many other black teas. The color of Nilgiri tea is of the most a classic amber-brown hue. They are beautifully fragrant, round in body, with undertones of red berries and honey. One Indian tea professional gave me an analogy I'll never forget, "The different teas of India reflect the character of the regions and the terrain where they're cultivated—Assam is a rough tea, Darjeeling most sophisticated and colonial in style, and the teas from Nilgiri are calm, approachable and easy to drink."

Tip: Great on ice.

Ceylon Ceylon teas have a unique, incisive flavor quality that totally says TEA, without any of the astringency or the malty dryness of Darjeeling and Assam teas. They're naturally slightly fruity. Imagine a classic black tea aroma, faint apricot in the taste and a hint of a caramel aftertaste. These teas don't lack in body, yet they're more mellow than bold. Ceylon teas have retained their traditional country name and are grown on the fertile, tropical island state of Sri Lanka. Located just off the southern tip of India, it's the fourth largest tea producing country in the world, and only about the size of the state of West Virginia. Five percent of the population works in the tea industry, and a similar fraction of the country's land is covered with beautiful tea plants. Sri Lanka now also produces green and white teas, which are as high in quality as their superb black teas.

Tip: Great for first time loose leaf tea drinkers.

Darjeeling Darjeeling is known as the Champagne of teas. The region of Darjeeling is beautiful and dramatically hilly, rising as high as 7,000 feet (2100 m) in the foothills of the Himalayas in a northern spur of India, about ten miles (16 km) from Nepal. Only at this altitude and microclimate is it possible to produce a slow growth of leaves with such delicacy. Darjeeling still maintains many of the tea traditions from its 19th century British roots, and tea is served in all its splendor every afternoon in the colonial estates. This tea is picked in three seasons or flushes each year—early and late spring and again in the fall—which produces three very distinctly recognizable styles of leaves from the same plants. The leaves from the early spring harvest are intense; you can almost feel that this flavor comes from a plant that has been dormant all winter and just couldn't wait to show its complex power. The term "muscatel," as in grapes, is used to describe the more mellow and round late spring and autumn harvest teas.

Tip: Use just a little less leaf, time and heat than you would for other black teas. (One LEVEL teaspoon [2 g], start with just UNDER 3 minutes, and use water at 195°F [90°C].) Also, Darjeeling cold brews very well. But don't tell anyone in Darjeeling this, they're pretty pure-bred traditionalists, and there's absolutely nothing cool about drinking your tea chilled there.

OOLONG

Iron Goddess of Mercy (*Ti Kuan Yin* or *Tie Guan Yin*) This truly is the goddess of Chinese oolongs, with fascinating aromas conjuring up images of spring flowers and intense toasty-sweet flavors with orchid floral notes. Tie Guan Yin's flavor just doesn't quit. You can steep these leaves four or five times. Its intensity is attributed to how the tea is processed, but also to its late spring harvest, which is said to bring out all the intensity built up during the long period of dormancy. Tie Guan Yin comes from China's Fujian Province, the birthplace of oolong teas, which go through a complex, manually intensive production. The region within Fujian where this oolong is grown is subtropical and has very rich soil. The terraced hillsides of tea plants are intensely beautiful, green and lush.

Tip: If you're thinking of going the Gongfu route, this is the tea you should try your skills out on. There's no other tea in our list that has as many different personalities through multiple steeps as Ti Guan Yin.

GREEN

Gunpowder Great name, right? It's not, however, a translation from its Chinese name *zhucha*, but maybe comes from one of several origins. This tea is tightly rolled in roughly shaped pellets, and in my mind, its dry leaves have both the metallic sheen and a slight aromatic tinge of gunpowder. Steeped up, it tastes thick and strong, with the characteristic Chinese green tea flavor undertones of grilled vegetables. This is a bold green tea, slightly reminiscent of charcoal and smoke, and seems best suited for drinking in fall and winter. Gunpowder tea leaves stay fresh longer than any other green tea leaves, thanks to their compressed form.

Tip: Go a bit short on steeping time the first time you try this tea. It's powerful, but if you approach it gently, you'll get to experience its best side.

Dragonwell (*Lung Ching* or *Long Jing*) The name is a literal translation from Long Jing, which as legend has it, was a well with thick water in it. After rainfalls, the lighter water on top would move around like a dragon. Are you into the romance of tea yet? Dragonwell is a beautiful tea with elegant long flat leaves. It steeps a clean yellow-green infusion, with fresh outdoor aromas to match the vibrant color of its leaves. The approach is sweet, of vegetables and grass, and the flavor buttery, with a slightly spicy and nutty aftertaste. Dragonwell is cultivated in the Westlake region of Zhejiang Province, China, an area of profound natural beauty and inspiration for designers, poets and painters.

Tip: Try going a little light on leaf quantity, you may be pleasantly surprised.

Clouds and Mist (*Yun Wu*) Yun Wu describes the mountains shrouded in mist where this tea is grown in Jiangxi Province, China. The aroma is slightly sweet and gently smoky. Yun Wu's flavor is well rounded, light and toasted because it's made with a pan fired process. The taste is reminiscent of sweet, gently roasted artichokes. The finish on this tea is soft, buttery and slightly nutty. Harvested in the spring from tender tea buds, clouds and mist tea has curly silver-green leaves. This tea, which has been cultivated for over 1,500 years, is even referred to in the famous 8th century Chinese treatise on natural medicine.

Tip: Re-steeps beautifully, so you can likely get two additional steeps from the same leaves. Add a full minute for each additional infusion.

Jasmine Green Tea Loose green tea or hand-rolled fresh tea buds are layered with jasmine flowers in the evening, when they open up and release their maximum perfume. This makes for an exquisitely scented jasmine green tea or jasmine pearls, as the rolled version is called. As they steep, the pearls open to unveil an almost intoxicating aroma. You might also see larger hand-tied flowering teas with a jasmine flower in the center. Many jasmine teas today are simply flavored and fragranced, making the process less labor-intensive. The green tea base for the leaf jasmine teas is often a Chinese *chun-mee* (smaller leaves) or green *pouchong* (larger leaves). The tasting profiles of jasmine teas vary depending on the process and the tea base, but the characteristic aroma of this tea is powerful and perseveres through the sweet and clean flavor of the tea.

Tip: Be careful not to exceed temperature or steeping time—or else go for the cold brew!

Sencha The most popular Japanese tea, making up over 75 percent of all of the country's tea production, is sencha. Japanese green teas are steam dried, so there's nothing roasted or charcoal-like about this tea. It's soft, yet bright on the palate, fresh and grassy in its aroma, and overall very refreshing to sip. Its flavors are sweetly algae and broth-like, with a little to some astringency. The soft and sweet approach of the tea lingers in your mouth. Sencha leaves are long, thin, flat and intense green in color. This tea is cultivated in all the tea-growing regions of Japan, and the top-dollar senchas come from Kagoshima prefecture in the southernmost part of the country.

Tip: You can steep sencha two to three times, and it makes a fantastic cold brew.

Gyokuro Gyokuro translates to "jade dew," descriptive of the color of its infusion. Umami is the taste sense that comes to mind when you sip this very fine pale cup of green tea, and aromas of the sea will dominate the nose. Gyokuro is very gentle in how it presents its flavors, but undeniably medium-bodied in how it feels in the mouth. The citrus and astringent aspects that you taste in sencha are not as present here; it's like pure, soft, sweet green tea on velvet. The leaves are very fine and needle-shaped and of a brilliant dark green color, which is due to its high chlorophyll content from spending the final part of its growing season in the shade. Most gyokuros are grown in Uji, which is between two of Japan's most revered historical and cultural centers, Kyoto and Nara, so you can imagine the care that goes into the production of this quintessential Japanese tea. You'll find that its price tag is reflective of its quality and stature in the tea world.

Tip: If you follow the steeping instructions exactly, this tea will make you feel like you're taking an exquisite plunge under the sea!

Hojicha The first thing you'll notice about this tea is its roasty aroma. Hojicha brews into a caramel, amber color with a slightly sweet, biscuity and nutty flavor. It's both soothing to drink this on cold winter days and refreshing to drink it iced. Hojicha is naturally lower in caffeine yet more robust in flavor than most other Japanese greens because of the roasting process. It's made using either sencha or the lower-grade bancha tea. This tea is a great first green tea for people who love espresso.

Tip: Very low in caffeine and rich in antioxidants.

Genmaicha If you've ever been served green tea in a sushi restaurant, it most likely was Genmaicha. Genmaicha is made from an everyday Japanese green tea called "bancha," combined with roasted brown rice, some grains of which have popped. The lovely vegetal green flavor, indicative of Japan's steaming process, is balanced by the nutty and wholesome flavor imparted by the roasted rice. The combination becomes an earthy tea that is as soothing to the soul as chicken noodle soup, making it a great gateway tea to pure Japanese green teas.

Tip: Super easy on the tummy.

WHITE

White Peony (*Bai Mu Dan* or *Pai Mu Dan*) This pure white tea from Fujian, China steeps into a golden-colored infusion. Its taste is sweet, slightly vegetal and nutty, with light notes of apricot or citrus. White Peony is smooth and easy to drink, with a lingering, buttery finish. The mouth-feel is round and fresh. It makes a satisfying iced tea, thanks to its natural sweetness. White teas have a subtle flavor that is closer to that of a fresh tea leaf than any other tea. Bai Mu Dan is large-leafed and fluffy. Less tea is used per serving, and when steeped for short periods of time, or cold brewed, it's very low in caffeine.

Tip: This tea cold brews fantastically.

21 WHOLE LEAF TEAS BY FLAVOR PROFILE

NAME	TYPE	CAFFEINE YIELD PER SERVING	ORIGIN	CHARACTER
Pu'erh	Pu'erh, or Dark Tea	High - one-half of coffee	China, Yunnan Province	Rich & Earthy
Assam	Black	High - one-third of coffee	India, Assam State	Assertive & Malty
Yunnan	Black	High - one-third of coffee	China, Yunnan Province	Honey & Peppery
Lapsang Souchong	Black	High - one-third of coffee	China, Yunnan Province	Smoky & Deep
English/Irish Breakfast	Black	High - one-third of coffee	India, China, and Sri Lanka	Bold & Full-Bodied
Earl Grey	Black	High - one-third of coffee	India, China, and Sri Lanka	Citrus & Smooth
Keemun	Black	High - one-third of coffee	China, Anhui Province	Toasty & Floral
Nilgiri	Black	High - one-third of coffee	India, Nilgiri State	Smooth & Fruity
Ceylon	Black	High - one-third of coffee	Sri Lanka	Crisp & Classic Black Tea Flavor
Darjeeling	Black, Darjeeling	High - one-third of coffee	India, West Bengal state	Bright & Muscatel
Iron Goddess of Mercy	Oolong	Medium - one-fourth of coffee	China, Fujian Province	Sweet Floral & Burnt Sugar
Gunpowder	Green	Medium - one-fifth of coffee	China, multiple regions	Bold & Lightly Smoky
Clouds & Mist	Green	Medium - one-fifth of coffee	China, Jiangxi Province	Muscatel & Artichoke
Dragonwell	Green	Medium - one-fifth of coffee	China, Zhejiang Province	Chestnut & Mellow
Jasmine Green	Green	Medium - one-fifth of coffee	China, multiple regions	Bright & Aromatic
Sencha	Green	Medium - one-fifth of coffee	Japan	Fresh Grass & Seaweed
Gyokuro	Green	Medium - one-fifth of coffee	Japan	Buttered Greens & Umami
Hojicha	Green	Medium - one-fifth of coffee	Japan	Sweet & Roasty
Genmaicha	Green	Medium - one-fifth of coffee	Japan	Nutty & Toasted
White Peony	White	Low - one-tenth of coffee	China, Fujian Province	Citrus & Buttery
Silver Needles	White	Low - one-tenth of coffee	China, Fujian Province	Delicate & Honeysuckle

← INCREASING BUZZ FACTOR →

Silver Needles (*Baihao Yinzhen*) Picked in the morning when these young tea buds are tightly enclosed in new leaves, this tea retains a silky, downy quality. It's true to its name, with long, straight silver-green buds. Not only is it an exquisite tea, but it also makes a great tool for actually observing tea bud anatomy. Silver Needles steeps into a beautiful light yellow-colored infusion. This is a tea about tenderness: delicate, classy and understated. When you sip it, you'll taste a soft, nourishing sweetness and eventually experience a similar sensation down your throat. Its flavor is naturally light, faint grassy-vegetal, with floral notes of honeysuckle, and a smooth, clean aftertaste. These exquisite tea buds are grown in China's Fujian Province.

Tip: Go gentle on the water temperature, making sure you don't exceed 170°F (75°C).

GOING BEYOND PURE TEA AND THE TEACUP

TEA LATTES

Between our national addiction to coffee and our love for milk, you're surely already familiar with coffee lattes. The very same foam can bring a creamy mellowness to your tea drink as well. Tea lattes are an attractive starter beverage for easing into tea for tea newbies, for first thing in the morning when some of us aren't yet ready to take on a straight tea yet. With very little work, and about $0.25–$0.35 in ingredients, you can blend up a latte every bit as tasty as the $4.00 one on the menu at your local café.

The Perfect Tea Latte

Yield: Two 12-ounce (355-ml) tea lattes

2 rounded tsp (4 g) whole leaf tea
16 oz (480 ml) water
¼ cup (60 ml) milk or milk substitute

Steep your favorite tea leaves in 16 ounces (480 ml) water at the right temp for your tea for as long as necessary to make an extra strong tea latte base. While tea is steeping, foam the milk, either with an automatic whisk or a milk steamer or foamer. Spoon the foamed milk, dividing evenly, into two 12-ounce (355-ml) mugs. Pour the tea brew over the foamed milk in each mug and serve immediately.

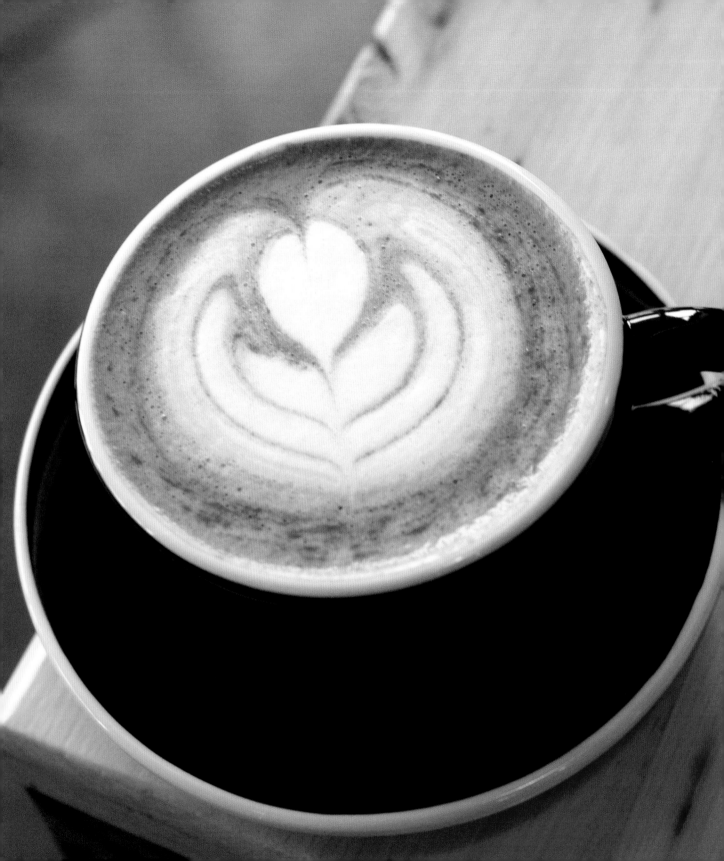

Matcha Green Tea Latte

Sip. Swoon. Sip some more. PS: Don't be fooled. Just so you know, this is one powerfully nourishing beverage. Each rounded ½ teaspoon of matcha gives you the antioxidant power of 5 pounds (2.3 kg) of wild blueberries or 50 servings of spinach.

Yield: One 10 ounce (300 ml) hot, or 16 ounce (480 ml) iced tea latte

¾ cup (180 ml) milk or milk substitute

½ tsp matcha green tea powder

¼ cup (60 ml) hot water (150°F [65°C])

Honey or agave, optional

Heat the milk or milk substitute. Briskly whisk the matcha into the hot water. Slowly add the milk or milk alternative and sweetener to taste. Blend well until super smooth. For an iced latte, just pour over a tall glass with ice to serve.

Five little tips to make your matcha latte crave-worthy:

1. Use the good stuff. The flavor of your latte is just as important as that of a ceremonial bowl of matcha. The splash of milk and sweetener won't mask a nasty green tea powder.

2. Use non-dairy milk. Maximize your stellar latte's benefits. Studies have shown that casein, the protein in milk, may interact negatively with the antioxidant activity of tea catechins in vivo, that is, in your gut. Personally, I love them best made with unsweetened almond milk.

3. Sweeten smartly and don't overdo it. Try using dates, vanilla, honey, agave, maple syrup or coconut palm sugar. Start with just a little bit. Getting the balance right between the flavor of the matcha and the sweet stuff is key. Using no sweetener is a valid option too!

4. Blend like mad. Have you ever seen Bulletproof coffee being made? They crank those suckers out on high speed in super-powered blenders. As sacrilegious and non-traditional as that can sound when dealing with your precious powder which spent its childhood carefully nurtured in shade, it works really well. You want it blended smooth and foamy. Your whisking arm can't compete with a 2 horsepower motor. This is also a great way to make it nice and hot.

5. Get creative. Try adding a fresh mint leaf or vanilla bean to the blender. Or try your matcha latte with a teaspoon (2 g) of cacao powder because two superfoods are better than one.

CHAI, 3 WAYS

One of the most popular tea lattes is the classic masala chai latte. "Chai" is the term for tea in India. In the western world, it most often refers to a strong, sweetened black tea mixed with milk and masala, a blend of ayurvedic spices believed to have protective effects on the immune system. The black tea base for chai is Assam, which many refer to as "the strong one." When you add milk to Assam tea, it turns a characteristic ruby color. You can easily make chai or a delicious and creamy chai latte with any tea type. As you adapt your recipe to your liking, you'll see that brewed fresh, it will be the best chai tea you've ever tasted.

Classic Spicy Masala Chai

Yield: 8 cups (1.9 L)

Spice Mix

1 tbsp (6 g) cloves

2 tsp (5 g) ground cardamom

2-inch (5-cm) piece fresh ginger, chopped

1 tsp (3 g) Tellicherry peppercorns

1 stick (or ½ tsp ground) cinnamon

1 tsp (1 g) broken bay leaf

4 cups (960 ml) fresh water, divided

2 tbsp (10 g) Assam black tea

¼ cup (80 ml) honey

4 cups (960 ml) milk, or milk alternative

Steep spice mix in 2 cups (480 ml) boiling water. Marinate overnight at room temperature. Strain out spices from marinade. Steep tea leaves in 2 cups (480 ml) boiling water for 5 minutes. Strain out tea leaves. Combine honey, strained spice mix marinade, tea and milk in a 2.5 to 3.5 quart (2 to 3 L) saucepan. Heat to hot simmer, stirring until honey is dissolved completely. Remove from heat, and serve immediately.

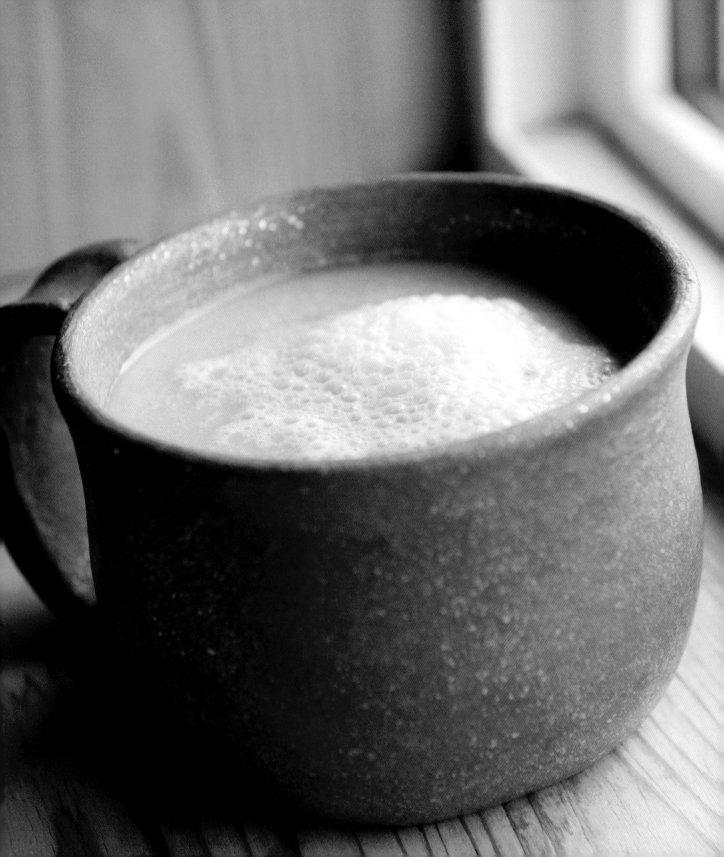

Red Chai

This sweet caffeine-free version of chai is a huge crowd pleaser. The rooibos blends beautifully with the spices, and maintains a beautifully smooth base to the drink. Great after dinner or as dessert on a chilly evening.

Yield: 8 cups (1.9 L)

1½ tsp (8 g) whole cloves

12 pods whole, or 1 tsp (2 g) ground cardamom

1 inch (2.5 cm) fresh ginger, chopped

½ tsp broken bay leaf

1 tsp (2 g) fennel seeds

1 tsp (2.5 g) Tellicherry peppercorns

1 stick or ½ tsp ground cinnamon

½ cup (50 g) red rooibos tea leaves

4 cups (960 ml) boiling water

½ cup (120 ml) honey

4 cups (960 ml) almond or soy milk

Add the first eight ingredients to 4 cups (960 ml) boiling water in a large mason jar. Cover and seal the jar. Allow it to cool and marinate at room temperature at least six hours or overnight to make the chai concentrate. Strain the spices and rooibos leaves out of the chai concentrate. You can keep this concentrate in the fridge for up to two days. When you're ready to make and serve your chai, heat the chai concentrate gently on the stove, over low to medium heat, and add honey. Allow the honey to dissolve completely, then add the milk. Heat the mixture just short of boiling, over medium-high heat. Remove it from the stove and serve immediately.

Green Tea Chai

Yield: 8 cups (1.9 L)

10 whole cloves

6 whole pods or 1 tsp (2 g) ground cardamom

2 inches (5 cm) fresh ginger, chopped

2 tsp (6 g) Tellicherry peppercorns

2 sticks, or 1 tsp (2 g) ground cinnamon

6 cups (1.4 L) fresh water

3 level tbsp (15 g) gunpowder green tea

½ cup (120 ml) honey

2 cups (480 ml) rice milk

Combine first 5 ingredients in a medium saucepan. Lightly crush the spices with the back of a spoon. Add water and bring to boil. Reduce heat and simmer gently for 15 minutes. Remove from heat and add tea leaves. Steep for 3 minutes. Strain out spices and tea leaves, and return liquid to pan. Add honey and stir until dissolved completely. Add rice milk, and bring to simmer. Remove from heat, and serve immediately.

HERBALS

The history of herbs and spices is even more ancient than that of tea. Herbal infusions are not tea, per se, as they don't come from the *Camellia sinensis* plant. They are hugely popular after-dinner and nighttime beverages, and naturally 100 percent caffeine-free. Many tea drinkers experience a variety of reputed benefits and many offer a sensory delight in great taste. People have turned to botanicals for centuries, either as refreshing, aromatic pick-me-ups or relaxing soothers, as well as for assistance with digestion, sleep and immunity. Herbal infusions include well-known flowering plants such as jasmine, chamomile, lavender and mint; herbs such as lemongrass and rosemary; florals such as rose, hibiscus and chamomile; roots such as ginger, ginseng and licorice; and other botanicals such as South African rooibos. Some exquisite tea blends include herbs and may even add seeds, berries, nuts and cocoa.

Herbs & Spices As with cooking, herbs and spices add variety and flavor to any cup. The possibilities are endless, but herbs such as peppermint, lemongrass and ginger root can all be enjoyed as a caffeine-free infusion or as an addition to your favorite tea.

Florals Many flowers go beyond your centerpiece to brew up a delicious and beneficial cuppa. Flowers such as jasmine, rose, chamomile and hibiscus all offer unique flavors and a slew of time-tested health benefits.

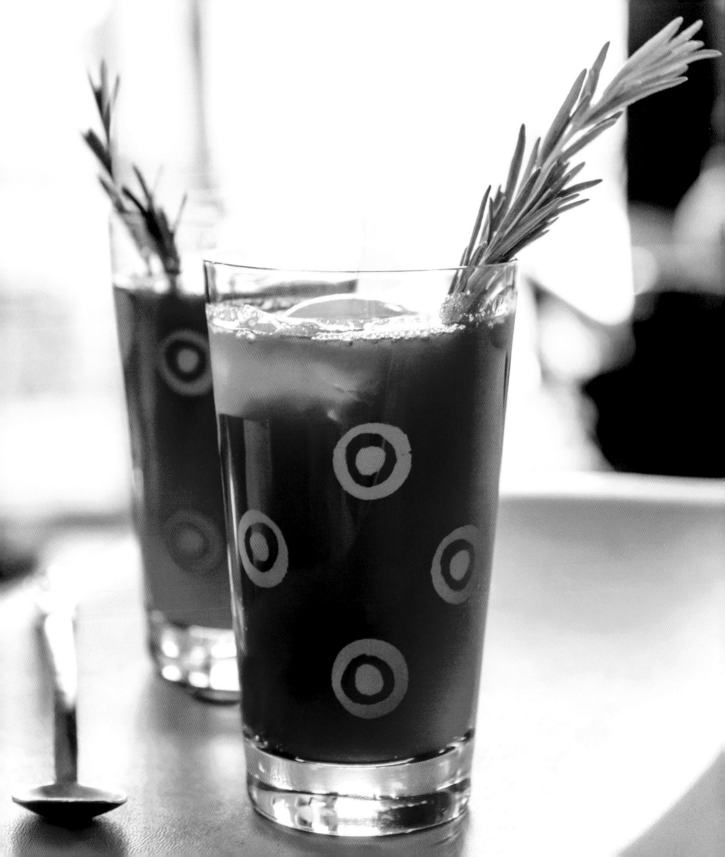

How to hot brew herbals: Infuse one heaping teaspoon (2 g) of herbs in 8 ounces (240 ml) of water at boiling point for 6 to 7 minutes. Strain out leaves.

How to cold brew herbals: Infuse one heaping teaspoon (2 g) of herbs in 16 ounces (480 ml) cold water for 10 to 15 minutes. Strain out leaves.

SOME HERBAL FAVORITES

Hibiscus This exotic, deep red herbal infusion steeps into a tart and thirst-quenching flavor, reminiscent of fresh cranberries. Grown throughout the tropics and subtropics of the world, hibiscus is a natural source of vitamin C and antioxidants and has been used to help manage minor hypertension. This is a beautifully refreshing tea, hot or cold brewed, and a perfect beverage year-round.

Serving tip: Try adding a sprig of mint or lavender, or sliced fresh ginger and lime juice to your hibiscus infusion.

Summer Hibiscus Cooler

Hibiscus petals make a great base for delicious mocktails. They're so colorful and flavorful you'll not miss the booze. Ginger beer is actually brewed and fermented. It has far less sugar and carbonation than ginger ale and a stronger ginger flavor. I originally made this recipe for a pregnant colleague who loves hibiscus and ginger, and we've all continued to enjoy it as a zippy summer drink ever since!

Yields two servings

2 heaping tsp (6 g) hibiscus
2 cups (480 ml) fresh, cool or room temperature water
1 slice fresh pineapple or ¼ cup (60 ml) pineapple juice
½ can (6 oz [175 ml]) ginger beer, chilled
Ice cubes
2 fresh rosemary sprigs

Make cold brewed hibiscus by allowing the hibiscus leaves to steep for 15 minutes in the water. Strain the leaves out and pour the hibiscus infusion into a cocktail shaker. Blend and strain the pineapple, if you're using the fresh stuff. Add the pineapple juice to the hibiscus and shake well.

Pour ginger beer into two glasses with ice, dividing evenly. Rub the rosemary sprigs between your hands vigorously for a few seconds to release their aroma and place into the glasses with the ginger beer. Divide the hibiscus tea between the two glasses. Stir gently and serve.

Chamomile This flowering plant in the daisy family has been brewed both fresh and dried for centuries. Chamomile is sought after to help relieve stress and induce feelings of relaxation. Recent studies indicates that chamomile may have a positive influence on weight loss. This could be directly related to its ability to promote calm and rest (both important to supporting healthy weight management), as well as its ability to help stimulate the production of gastric juices. Caffeine-free.

Sparkling Tea

Sparkling tea is basically just a tea variation on natural soda pop. Tea infuses in sparkling water just like it cold brews in water. Using different teas and herbals, you can make sparkling teas in an array of different flavors and colors. If you want to make it more fancy, you can add a squeeze of lemon, sprig of lavender, mint or a touch of simple syrup. I throw the tea leaves right in the bottle, and then serve the sparkling tea right from the soda bottle, through a filter which screws onto the plastic bottle. My favorite tea flavors for sparkling are chamomile, mint and aged white and green teas. These are perfect for summer and perfect for kids.

Yields four 8-ounce (240-ml) servings

32 oz (960 ml) unflavored sparkling water, in a bottle

3–4 tsp (6–8 g) loose leaf tea or herbals

Ice cubes

Open the bottle of sparkling water, and pour out ½ cup (120 ml) from the bottle. Add the tea or herbal leaves to the bottle with a narrow spoon or funnel. You can easily improvise a funnel with a sheet of paper. Screw the lid back onto the bottle, and shake gently to ensure the leaves are infusing all the water in the bottle. Wait 10 to 15 minutes for the leaves to cold brew. Open the bottle back up and pour your sparkling tea through a filter or a strainer into four glasses filled with ice, dividing evenly.

Great combos to try are:

Chamomile with an added sprig of lavender or mint

Green sencha tea with fresh lemon

Aged white tea with a touch of honey or agave

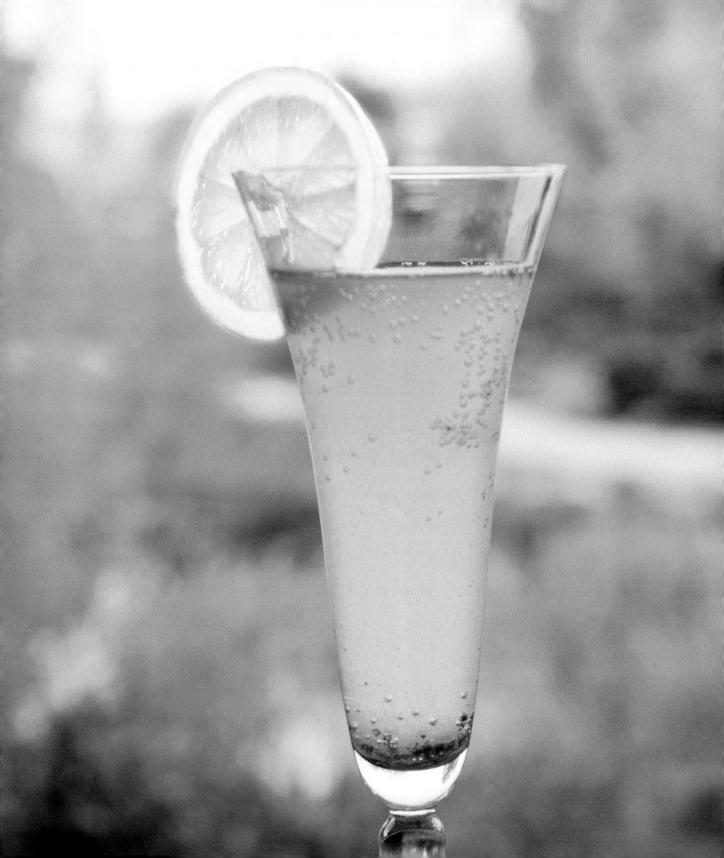

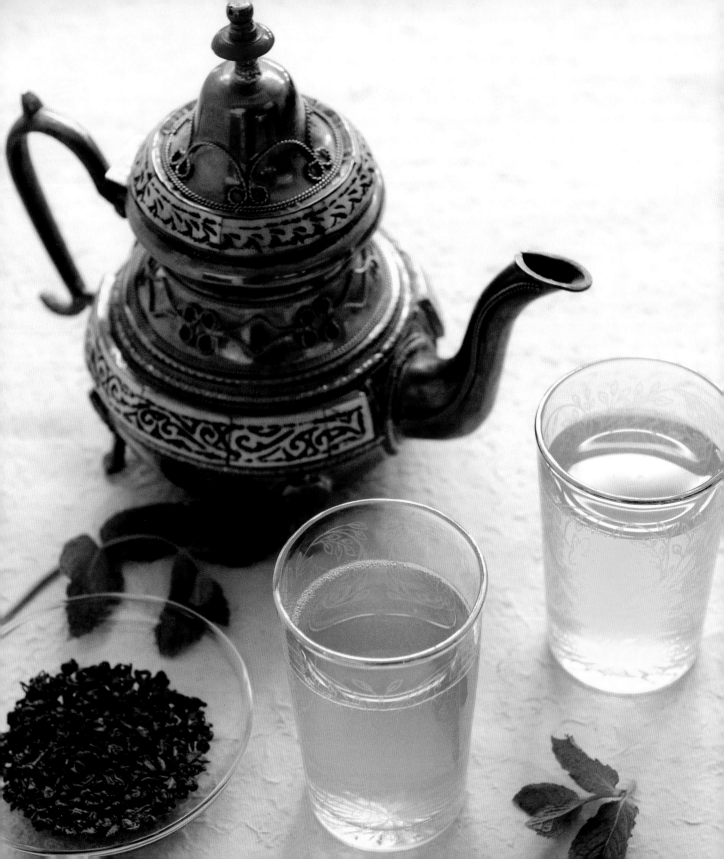

Mint A native of the Mediterranean, peppermint leaves were used to crown luminaries in ancient Greece and Rome. Peppermint continues to be revered for its strong and refreshing aroma and sweet and peppery taste. A freshly brewed cup may aid your digestion at the end of a meal. Spearmint tea is a little milder and sweeter in flavor than peppermint. It takes its name from its leaves, which resemble the shape of the blade of a spear.

Unsweetened Moroccan Mint

Take a bottle of this refreshing and rehydrating green tea with you on your next warm or cold weather hike. It will put a smile on your face and make you feel restored, while replenishing your body with antioxidants and giving you a gentle long-term caffeine boost. This version of Moroccan Mint tea without any sugar is not the authentic preparation, but it's even more drinkable than the sugary-sweet version you'd be served in Marrakech. You can drink a lot more of it when it's zero calories, and being sugar-free, it makes a far more effective thirst-quencher.

Yield: 2 cups (480 ml)

16 oz (480 ml) fresh water at boiling point
½ cup (about ½ ounce [15 g]) loosely packed fresh mint leaves
2 rounded tsp (6 g) gunpowder green tea

Bring the water to a boil and add the mint leaves. Allow them to steep uncovered for 3 minutes. Add the gunpowder green tea leaves to the mint and water, and let it all steep for three minutes longer. Strain out the mint and tea leaves. Serve hot, or chill, if desired.

Rooibos (red tea, red bush or honey bush tea) These needle-like leaves hail from the rugged Cederberg mountains of South Africa. Rooibos is touted for numerous health benefits, including anti-allergen effects, protection against the sun's UV rays and promoting a healthy immune system (rooibos has flavonoids). Rooibos infuses into a deep, rich, red infusion containing a multitude of minerals such as iron, potassium and calcium. This powerful red herbal has a sweet and earthy aroma, reminiscent of fresh tobacco, and exceptionally smooth flavor.

Serving Tip: Try this one iced. With its many minerals and lack of caffeine, rooibos is a fantastically effective drink for keeping hydrated.

Capetown Fog Tea Latte

Yield: Two 12 ounce (355 ml) tea lattes

2 tsp (5 g) rooibos tea leaves

16 oz (480 ml) water, at boiling point

¼ cup (60 ml) milk or milk substitute

Steep the rooibos in water for 8 minutes to make an extra strong tea latte base. While the rooibos is steeping, foam the milk, either with an automatic whisk or a milk steamer. Spoon the foamed milk, dividing evenly, into large mugs. Pour the rooibos brew over the milk in each mug and serve immediately.

Caffeinated Black Tea Variation: London Fog

Follow the same recipe as for the Capetown Fog Tea Latte above, but substitute black Earl Grey tea for the rooibos, and steep the tea for only five minutes. You can make your London Fog even more uplifting by adding a sprig of lavender to the finished beverage or by using a lavender Earl Grey tea base. Cheers!

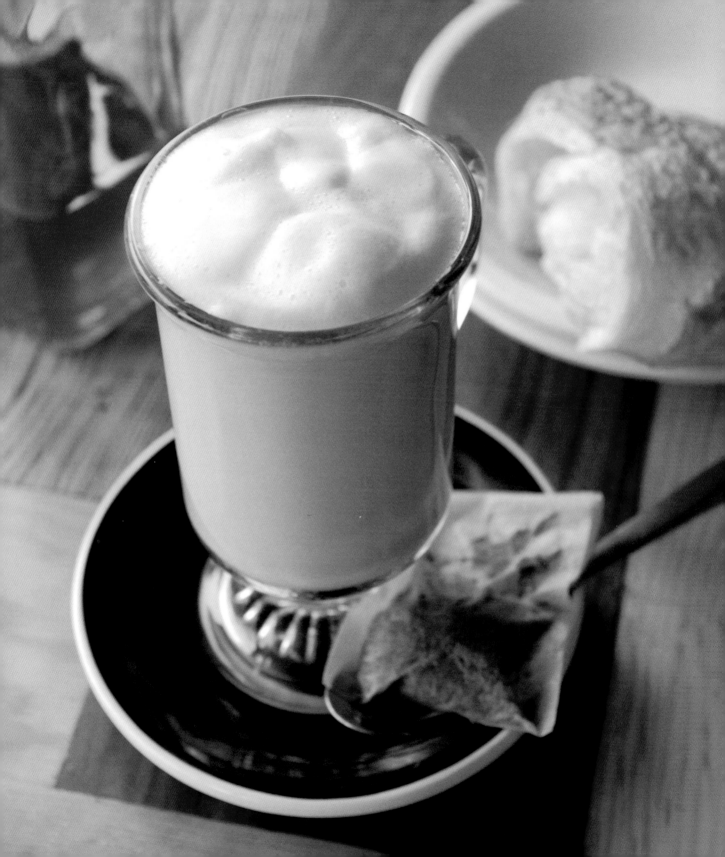

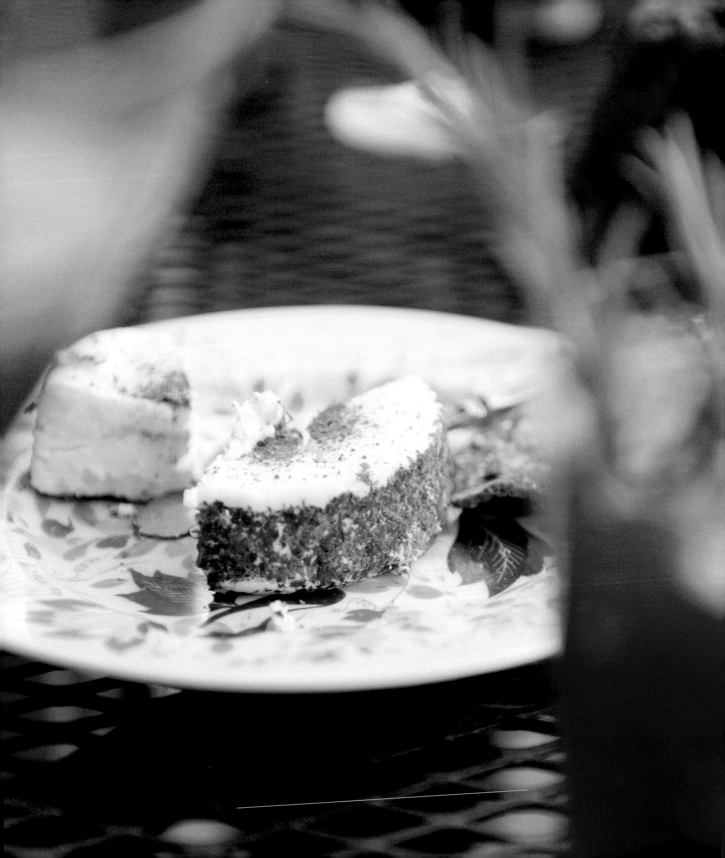

Chapter 11

EAT IT, CANCER

EAT GOOD FOOD. FEEL REAL GOOD.

If the last chapter left you feeling like you'd never be able to get enough tea into your day, this chapter offers some more ways to enjoy the magical tea leaf by adding it to your food. Food is so damn important. It nourishes us, soothes us and brings us together. It's one of life's great pleasures. Health care practitioners are recognizing more and more the immunizing and healing power of nutrition in regard to cancer and many other major diseases. The best medicine is real food. And there are few things as pure as tea in our diets.

In this chapter we present ten recipes, plus a few options for snacks, all of which pack a great antioxidant punch. It may seem like matcha madness has set in here, so let me explain! There are many beautiful tea recipes and cookbooks that evoke the spirit of tea and the essence of its many flavors. However, many of those don't actually give you much per serving in terms of tea polyphenols. All of the recipes featured here have been developed to taste yummy and be wholly satisfying and also to ensure that they actually provide ample tea benefits with each serving. You can substitute any one of these in your daily quest of those five antioxidant-rich cups (1.2 L) of tea.

Drinking enough tea every day to make an impact on your health may feel challenging at first, but once this tweak to your daily routine becomes your new norm, it's only a matter of time before your body will feel amazing and naturally ease its own way into additional anti-cancer behaviors. Tea can be a most loyal and supportive companion to you on this quest to getting to your peak state of immunity. Consistency in your anti-cancer actions is what cancer will hate the most, so just keep in mind that every day is the most important day to do some small step to keep cancer at bay.

Now let's go eat some tea.

Green Matcha Juice and Tonic

This juicing recipe will get you to re-think your drink. As a shot, it can be pretty intense for those who aren't used to juicing greens, but damn, it will wake you up and make you feel good! If you want to sweeten it up a bit, just add a juiced green apple. If you're looking to ease into the intensity of the fresh greens, the tonic option, with sparkling water added, is a great way to go.

Yield: 4 ounces (120 ml) juice or 12 ounces (350 ml) sparkling tonic

½-inch (1-cm) ginger root

½ cucumber, cut in 2 equal pieces

Pinch of cilantro

½ lemon or lime with rind

1 tsp (2 g) matcha

Chilled sparkling water (optional)

Juice the ginger root, followed by ¼ cucumber, then the cilantro, lemon or lime, and finally, the remaining ¼ cucumber. Whisk the matcha into the juice and serve immediately, in a small juice glass. If making a tonic, add the sparkling water to whatever volume or strength you like, and serve in a tall glass.

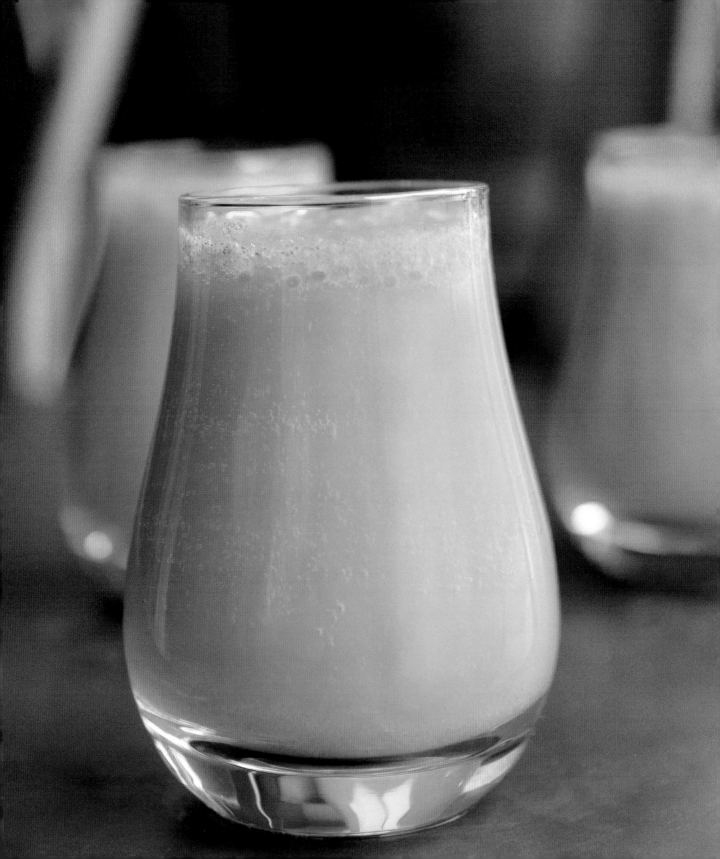

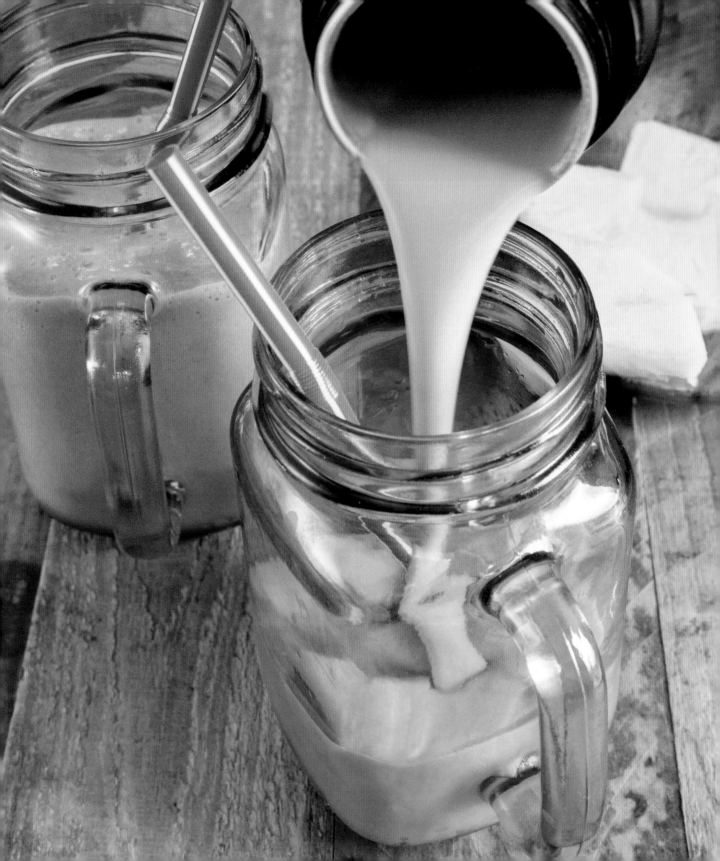

Organic Faux Piña Colada

You can choose to make the most of your matcha ingredient for flavor, or hide everything, including its borderline neon color. This drink succeeds in doing both. Its Piña Colada flavor is so believable, you could even serve this as a mocktail. It's also fresh and healthy enough that you can feel good about starting your day off with it.

Yields two 8-ounce (240-ml) smoothies

6 oz (180 ml) carrot-orange juice

2 oz (60 ml) unsweetened coconut milk

6 oz (170 g) frozen mango pieces

2 oz (60 g) frozen pineapple pieces

1 tsp (2 g) matcha

Optional—grated ginger root (small amount)

Add all the ingredients to a high-speed blender. Run at medium-high speed, or smoothie setting, until blended smooth. You can serve these in medium-size glasses as a breakfast smoothie. Alternatively, they can be served in large margarita or martini glasses as a healthy mocktail.

Matcha Morning Bowl

This concept takes the matcha smoothie and brings it to a whole new level. Don't shy away from trying interesting choices as toppings to add texture and flavors. The electric green color of matcha is amplified in this breakfast bowl, which will make any contrasting toppings look stellar. Try blueberries, strawberries, raspberries and blackberries, shredded coconut or granola. My favorite combo is with shaved coconut and blueberries.

Yields two 8-ounce (225 g) morning bowls

¼ avocado

¼ banana

1 cup (40 g total) each, loosely packed fresh parsley and cilantro

¼-inch (5-mm)-thick slice of organic lime (with skin)

1-inch (2.5 cm) fresh ginger root, peeled and sliced

8 oz (240 ml) coconut water

1 tsp (2 g) matcha

¾ cup (180 g) frozen pineapple pieces

4–5 ice cubes, as needed, for desired texture

Granola, or other optional toppings

Place all the ingredients, except the ice cubes and toppings, into a high-speed blender. Purée, slowly increasing to a medium speed, until smooth. Add the ice cubes, one by one, and blend until the mixture is at your desired consistency for a breakfast bowl—it should be similar to the texture of yogurt. Divide into 2 cereal bowls, add your favorite toppings and serve immediately.

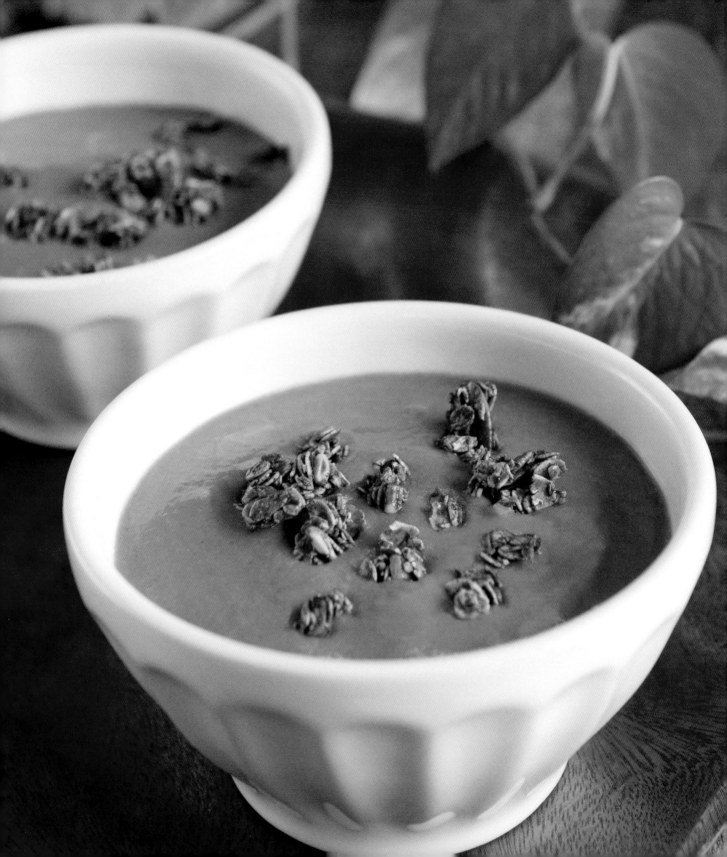

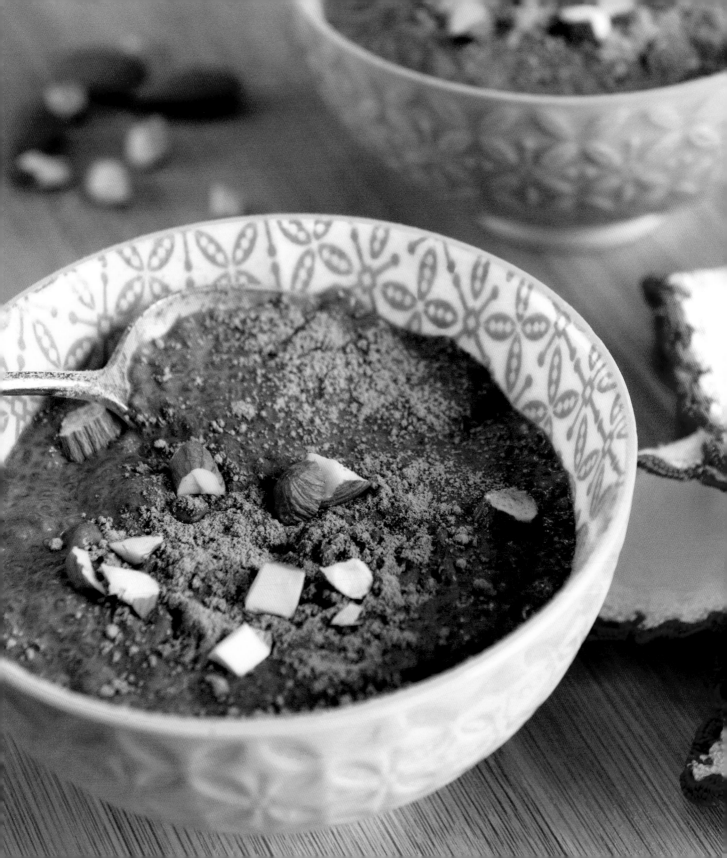

Matcha Chia Pudding with Cacao

This nutritious breakfast treat is straightforward and effortless to make. You can prep it the day before, and overnight the chia seeds will expand into a tasty, chewy tapioca-like pudding. With toppings or without, it's filling and delicious. You can make a few individual servings at a time in mini mason jars—they'll keep in the fridge for up to three days, so you can have your breakfast ready to go all week long.

Yields 2–3 Servings

2 cups (480 ml) almond or coconut milk

2 tbsp (30 ml) maple syrup

1 tsp (4 g) vanilla extract

1½ tsp (3 g) matcha

1 tbsp (7.5 g) cacao powder (you can leave this out if you are just craving the matcha pudding without any cacao!)

6 tbsp (60 g) chia seeds

Optional: fresh fruit and berries, nuts, seeds, cacao nibs, honey or maple syrup

Whisk or blend everything except the chia seeds and other garnishes together. Place the chia seeds in a medium-size bowl, and pour the blended mixture over them, stirring well to mix. Cover and let sit overnight in the fridge. Note: You can also place these into smaller mason jars before refrigerating, to make individual servings. To serve, spoon the pudding into cereal bowls. You can dress it up with raspberries, nuts and flax or hemp seeds. You can also drizzle with more maple syrup or sprinkle with cacao nibs.

Morning Glory Oatmeal

Every spoonful of this oatmeal is like a taste of sweet summer sunshine. The creamy consistency of this overnight creation highlights the sweeter, gentler side of matcha. It takes just a few minutes to prep and develops its nice flavor and texture without any cooking. Ideally, it should be left to chill in the fridge overnight before serving. It will keep in the fridge for up to four days. If you're really pressed for time after your morning tea, you can just put a beautiful spill-proof jar of oatmeal in your bag and make everyone at work envious of your delectable morning treat!

Yields 2-3 Servings

1 cup (80 g) rolled oats

1 tbsp (7 g) ground flax seeds

1 very ripe banana, mashed

½ cup (120 g) applesauce

1 cup (240 ml) unsweetened almond milk or coconut milk

1 large carrot, grated

2 tsp (4 g) matcha

1 tbsp (15 ml) honey

1 tsp (2.5 g) cinnamon

¼ cup (30 g) chopped walnuts

Optional: dollop of Greek yogurt and maple syrup, for topping

Stir the rolled oats and ground flax seeds into mashed banana and applesauce. Gently stir in the milk and all other ingredients, except walnuts and optional toppings. Mix everything together well. Spoon into a single large mason jar, or into four individual serving mason jars. Cover and let sit for at least four hours in the fridge. When serving, top with walnuts. You can also top this with Greek yogurt or drizzle with maple syrup.

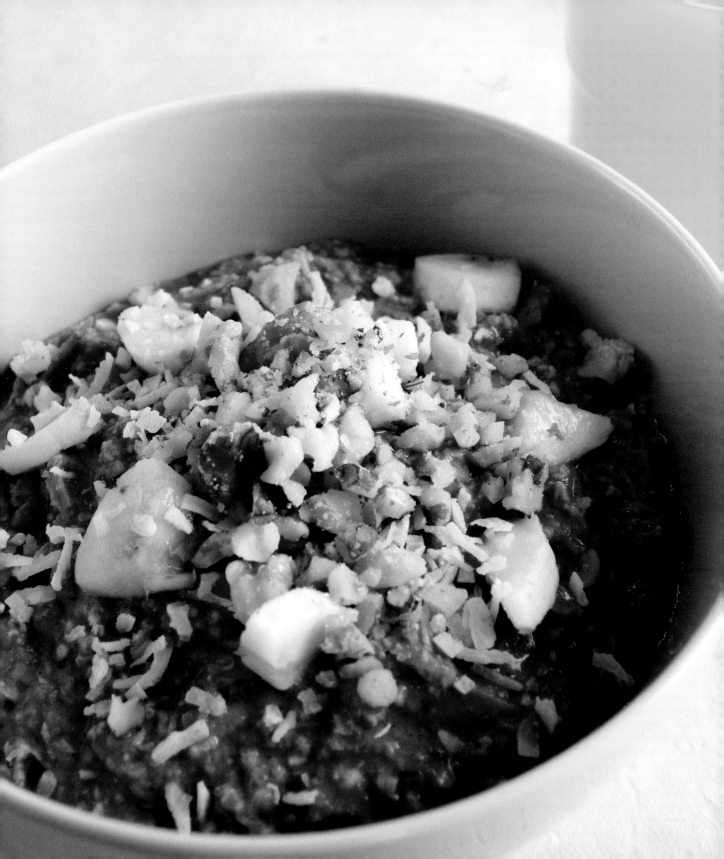

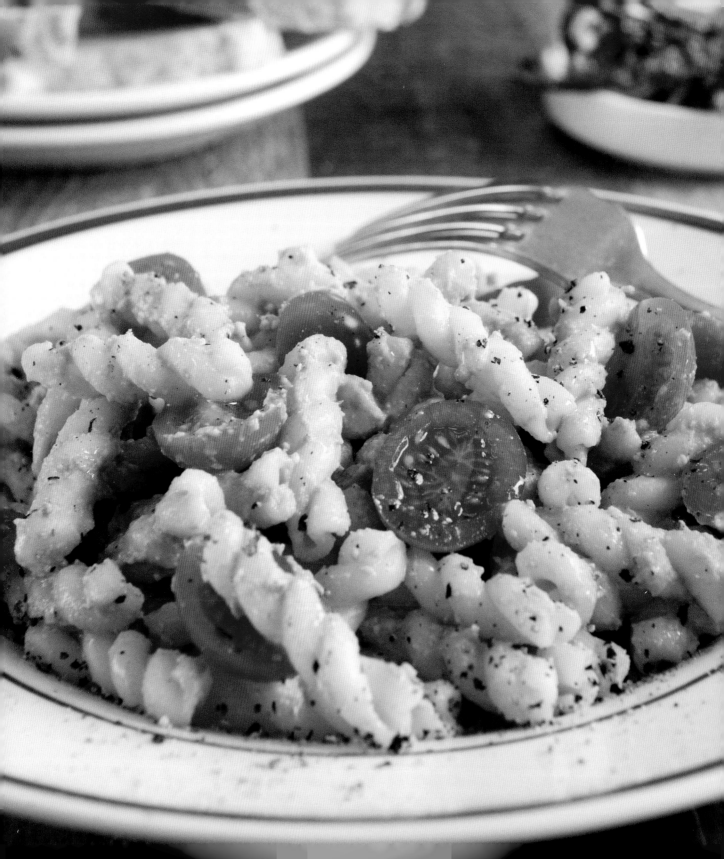

SAVORY RECIPES

Vegan Matcha Alfredo

Vegan Alfredo recipes have become wildly popular, using cauliflower, garlic and almond milk as an easy and healthy base. Matcha enhances this recipe beautifully, adding a green vegetal component to the blended mix of flavors. Alongside the cashews and nutritional yeast, you won't even find yourself missing the cheese, but non-vegans should feel free to add some real parmesan or Pecorino Romano to the finished dish.

This sauce can also be used to make a flavorful and intriguing green pizza sauce. Just spread it over a ready-to-bake pizza crust, and top with fresh spinach, shredded carrots, raisins, walnuts and mozzarella. Bake according to the instructions for your pizza crust.

Yields 6 Servings

1 whole cauliflower, chopped up into 8-12 pieces

2 cloves minced garlic

1 cup (150 g) roasted cashews

1 tbsp (15 ml) extra virgin olive oil

2 tbsp + 1 tsp (20 ml) lemon juice

½ cup (120 ml) unsweetened almond milk

¾ cup (100 g) nutritional yeast

1 tbsp (6 g) matcha

½ tsp onion powder

¼ tsp garlic powder

1 tsp (6 g) salt

Ground pepper to taste

1 lb (450 g) package dry pasta

2 pints (500 g) organic cherry tomatoes

Optional: Parsley or basil, black olives cured in olive oil, for garnish

Steam the cauliflower for 8-10 minutes until tender, making sure it's fully cooked, but not falling apart. Combine all the ingredients except pasta, tomatoes and optional garnishes in a food processor, and pulse in short spurts, until creamy. Add more almond milk, or olive oil if needed, until it gets to a sufficiently creamy consistency. Taste the sauce for seasoning, and add salt and pepper, if necessary. Slice the cherry tomatoes in half and put aside. Cook your pasta according to the directions on the package. Drain, and immediately pour the sauce over the cooked pasta, mixing gently until all the pasta is nicely coated. Add the sliced tomatoes and fold in gently. You can add any of these for garnish: parsley, basil or black cured olives.

Matcha Pesto, 2 ways

Pesto means "to pound" in Italian. We'll pulverize ours, thank you. The result is still super green, zesty, raw, healthy and delicious. In my home, appetizers are often impromptu and made quickly. This is a convenient way for you to work that extra serving of tea into your day, when unexpected guests come by!

Pesto Appetizer

This pesto is best served as an appetizer at room temperature. Place it in a serving dish and top with ¼ cup (50 g) chopped pistachios. It's great fun to serve this flavorful app and have people marvel at how tasty it is—only to tell them it's made with green tea. Even pesto snobs will find this unique recipe to their liking! It stands well on its own served with bread sticks.

Yields about 1 cup (240 ml) (serves 6-8)

1 tbsp (6 g) matcha

2 tsp (10 ml) water

3 tbsp (45 ml) freshly squeezed lemon juice

½ cup (120 ml) extra virgin olive oil

1 cup (20 g) each, loosely packed fresh parsley and sage

1 cup (125 g) raw shelled pistachios

6 cloves peeled garlic

¼ tsp sea salt, or more to taste

Combine all the ingredients in a food processor and pulse repeatedly until chopped coarse, like crunchy peanut butter. If it's too crumbly in texture, add a touch more olive oil.

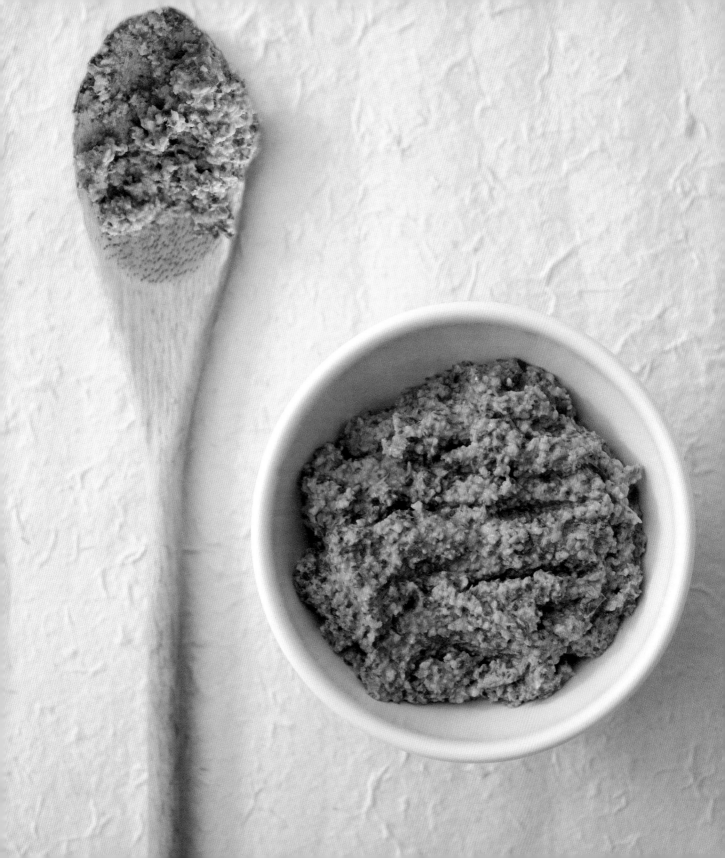

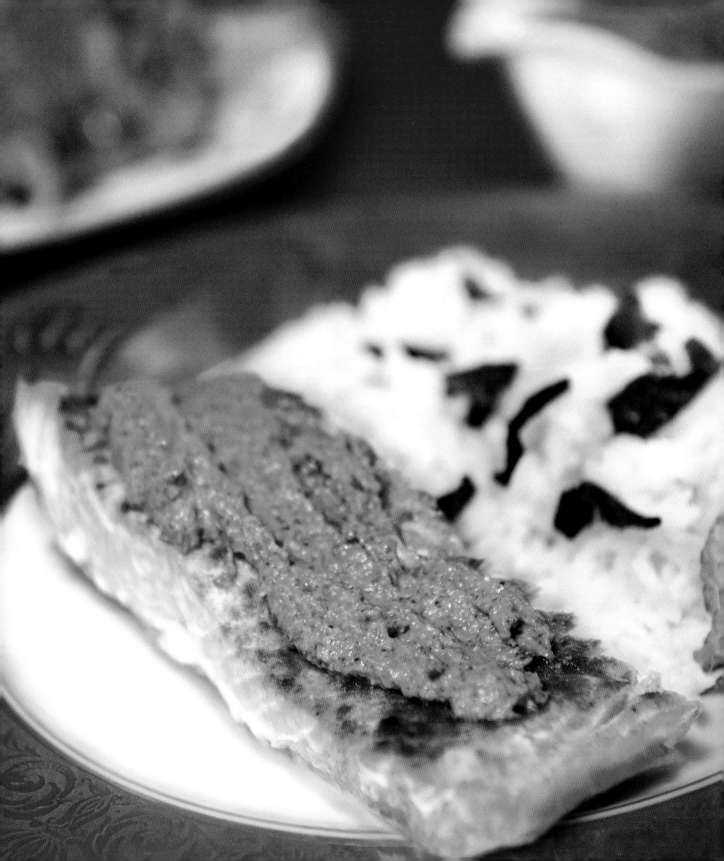

Pesto Sauce

This saucy pesto is equally delicious served warm or at room temperature. As an appetizer, it pairs super well with crudités, goat cheese, bread, toasts or pita chips. Thanks to its creamy nature, it also makes a delightful sauce for salmon, pasta, spiralized veggie "pasta" or a quinoa salad. My favorite way to serve it is tossed with zucchini pasta, with a poached egg on top.

Yields about 1 cup (240 ml) (serves 6-8)

1 tbsp (6 g) matcha

1 tbsp (15 ml) water

3 tbsp (45 ml) freshly squeezed lemon juice

½ cup (120 ml) extra virgin olive oil

1 cup (20 g) each, loosely packed fresh parsley and mint

1 cup (125 g) raw shelled walnuts

4 cloves peeled garlic

¼ tsp sea salt, dash of white pepper (optional)

Combine all the ingredients in a food processor, and pulse with longer repetitions until it's just barely creamy. If the texture isn't to your liking, try adding a few drops of water or lemon juice, until you reach the desired consistency.

Matcha Salad Dressing

Enjoy this healthy and delicious dressing over your favorite mixed green salad, steamed greens or quinoa. It's even great on sliced strawberries!

Yields 2-4 servings

1 tsp (2 g) matcha

2 tbsp (30 ml) rice vinegar

1½ tsp (8 ml) each, honey and lemon juice

¼ cup (60 ml) extra virgin olive oil

½ tsp shallots, finely diced

Sea salt and freshly ground black pepper

Stir matcha vigorously for 1 minute into rice vinegar. Gradually add honey and lemon juice, continuing to stir rapidly. Slowly add the olive oil, while stirring continuously. Mix in shallots and season with sea salt and freshly ground black pepper, to taste.

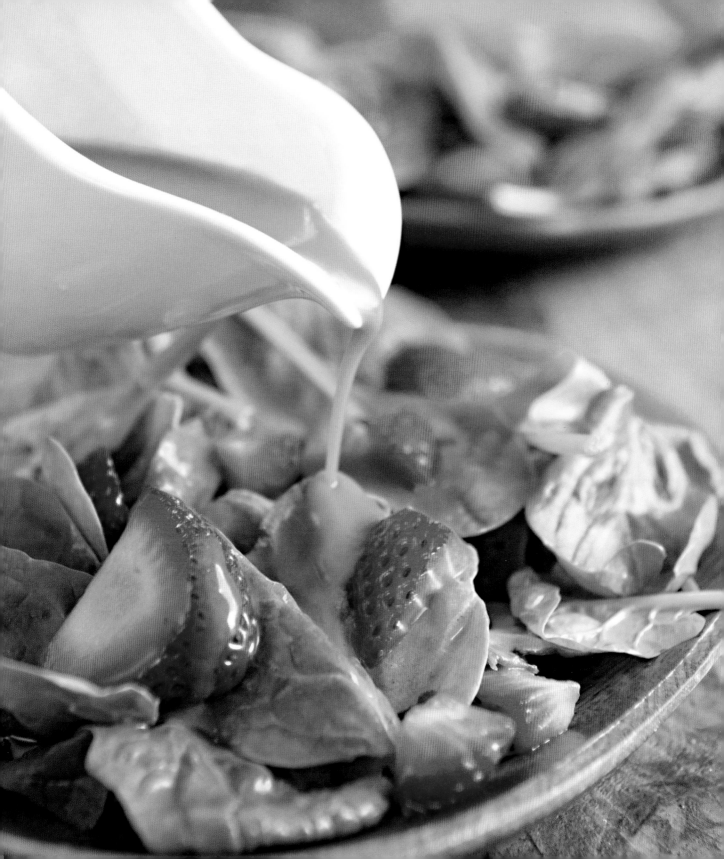

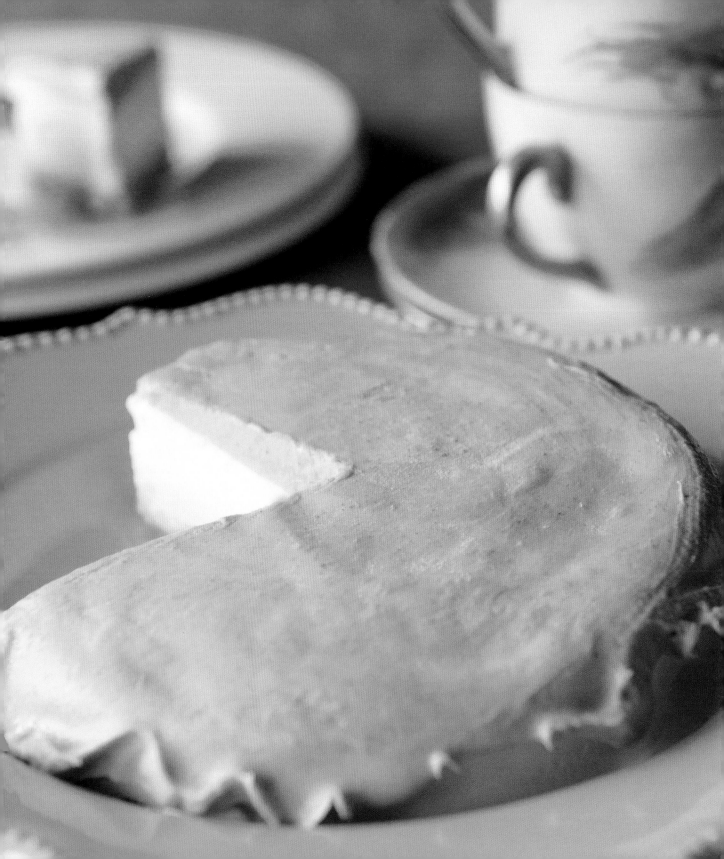

SWEETS

Matcha Key Lime Cheesecake

You'll be thanking the plants once you taste this sinfully delicious vegan cheesecake.

Yields 12 servings

Crust
1 cup (175 g) packed pitted dates
1 cup (140 g) raw almonds
Pinch of sea salt

Filling
1½ cups (225 g) raw cashews, soaked overnight
⅓ cup (70 g) coconut oil, melted
½ cup + 2 tbsp (150 g) full-fat coconut milk
¼ cup (60 ml) key lime juice
¼ cup (60 ml) agave
2 tbsp (12 g) matcha

Garnish
½–1 tsp (1–2 g) matcha

To make the crust, make sure the dates are soft. If they aren't, soak them for 10 minutes, and then pat them dry, before you add to the food processor. Place the almonds into a food processor and pulse until they've made a mealy texture. Remove this almond meal and put the dates into the food processor. Pulse these until they form a well-blended ball. Reintroduce the almond meal, add the sea salt and pulse both components together, until they're nicely incorporated.

To make the filling, place all filling ingredients except the matcha into a food processor and blend them until creamy. Set aside about ¾ of this mixture. Blend the matcha into the remaining filling in the food processor. Lightly grease a springform pan with coconut oil, and press the raw crust mixture into the base of the pan. Pour the filling mixture without matcha onto the crust and place the pan in the freezer until it's just slightly set—about 30 to 60 minutes. Remove the pan with cheesecake from freezer and pour the rest of the filling, with the matcha blended in, on top. You can marbleize this green portion into the cheesecake, or just keep it as the top layer. Place the pan with the cheesecake back in the freezer, overnight, until it's well frozen. One half hour before you plan on serving it, remove the cheesecake from the freezer and its springform pan. Garnish with some more matcha powder, slice and serve.

Matcha Truffles

Enjoy the healthy goodness! These visually stunning treats are vegan, raw and yummy.

Yields about 12 truffles, or 2-4 dessert servings

1 cup (140 g) almonds

1 cup (175 g) pitted dates tightly packed

1 tsp (2 g) matcha

Pinch of salt

Optional Toppings

Unsweetened baking cocoa

Melted chocolate of your choice

A mix of matcha & flaxseed meal

Shredded coconut, optionally dusted with matcha

Add the almonds to a high speed blender or food processor and process until mealy. Remove this almond meal and put the dates into the food processor. Pulse these until they form a well-blended ball. Add the almond meal back in, then the matcha, a pinch of salt and pulse until it's all well incorporated. Now it's time to make your truffles. Form them into individual balls by scooping a spoonful of the mixture at a time and rolling quickly between your hands. To add the outermost layer, roll the truffles in the toppings of your choice. Refrigerate for at least 2 hours before serving.

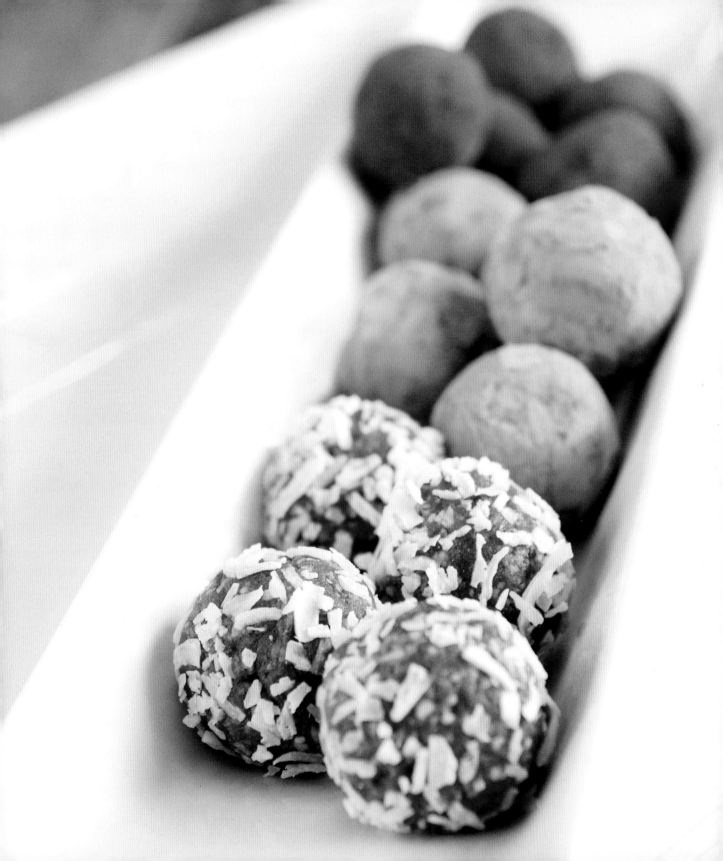

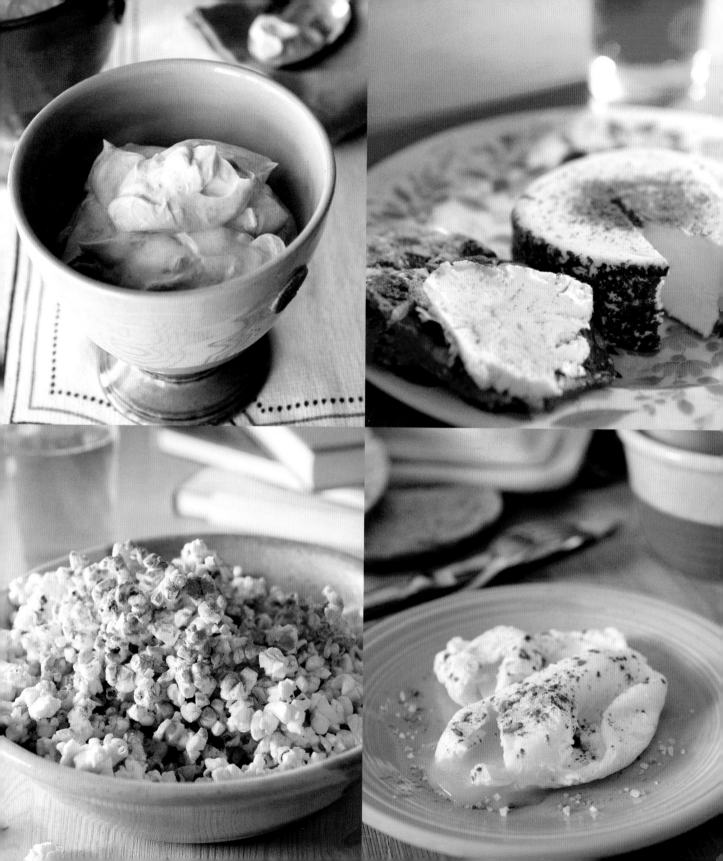

SNACKS

Ten Ways to Snack on Tea

You can easily sneak several doses of fresh green tea into snacks and mini meals throughout your day. Here are some quick and yummy ways to add that ½ teaspoon matcha serving.

* Stir it into yogurt

* Add it to your favorite green smoothie recipe

* Mix with 1½ teaspoons (4 g) nutritional yeast and sprinkle on your popcorn

* Mix with a ½ teaspoon rock salt and season your eggs

* Mix with a ½ teaspoon rock salt and sprinkle on goat cheese and crackers

* Mix it with extra virgin olive oil, sesame oil or soy sauce in cooking

* Blend it into your salad dressing

* Blend it with your maple syrup, on just about anything

* Blend it into your coconut, pistachio, vanilla or dark chocolate gelato

* Mix it with other superfoods, such as chia seeds, quinoa, almonds or even cacao

REFERENCES

CHAPTER 1

Anand, Preetha, Ajaikumar B. Kunnumakara, Chitra Sundaram, Kuzhuvelil B. Harikumar, Sheeja T. Tharakan, Oiki S. Lai, Bokyung Sung, and Bharat B. Aggarwal. "Cancer is a Preventable Disease that Requires Major Lifestyle Changes." *Pharmaceutical Research* 25(9) (2008): 2097–2116.

Mukhtar H, Ahmad N. "Tea polyphenols: Prevention of cancer and optimizing health." *American Journal of Clinical Nutrition* 71(6 Suppl) (2000): 1698S–1702S.

Cabrera C, Giménez R, López MC. "Determination of tea components with antioxidant activity." *Journal of Agricultural and Food Chemistry* 51(15) (2003): 4427–4435.

Lobo V, A. Patil, A. Phatak, and N. Chandra. "Free radicals, antioxidants and functional foods: Impact on human health." *Pharmacognosy Review* 4(8) (2010): 118–126.

Chaturvedula, Venkata Sai Prakash and Indra Prakash. "The aroma, taste, color and bioactive constituents of tea." *Journal of Medicinal Plants Research* 5(11) (2011): 2110–2124.

McKay, DL and JB Blumberg. "The role of tea in human health: an update." *Journal of the American College of Nutrition* 21(1) (2002): 1–13.

Katiyar, SK, and H. Mukhtar. "Tea in chemoprevention of cancer: epidemiologic and experimental studies." *International Journal of Oncology* 8 (1996): 221–38.

Lodish, H., et al. *Molecular Biology of the Cell, 5th ed.* (New York, Freeman, 2004)

Dreosti, IE, MJ Wargovich, and CS Yang. "Inhibition of carcinogenesis by tea: the evidence from experimental studies." *Critical Reviews in Food Science and Nutrition* 37 (1997): 761–70.

Kohlmeier, L, KGC Weterings, S Steck, and FJ Kok. "Tea and cancer prevention: an evaluation of the epidemiologic literature." *Nutrition and Cancer* 27 (1997): 1–13.

Hollman, PC, LB Tijburg, and CS Yang. "Bioavailability of flavonoids from tea." *Critical Reviews in Food Science and Nutrition* 37 (1997): 719–38.

Sadzuka, Y, T Sugiyama, and S. Hirota. "Modulation of cancer chemotherapy by green tea." *Clinical Cancer Research* 4 (1998): 153–6.

Wright, SC, J Zhong, and JW Larrick. "Inhibition of apoptosis as a mechanism of tumor promotion." *Federation of American Societies for Experimental Biology Journal* 8 (1994): 654–60.

Ahmad, N, DK Feyes, AL Nieminen, et al. "Green tea constituent epigallocat-echin-3-gallate and induction of apoptosis and cell cycle arrest in human carcinoma cells." *Journal of the Nationall Cancer Institute* 89 (1997): 1881–6.

Harbowy, Matthew E., and Douglas A. Balentine. "Tea Chemistry." *Critical Reviews in Plant Sciences* 16(5) (1997): 415–480.

Li, S, CY Lo, MH Pan, C Laic, and CT Hoa. "Black tea: chemical analysis and stability." *Food & Function* 1 (2013): 10–18.

Reygaert, WC. "The antimicrobial possibilities of green tea." *Frontiers in Microbiology* 5 (2014): 434.

CHAPTER 2

USDA Database for the Flavonoid Content of Selected Foods, Release 2.1. (2007).

Wu, X, GR Beecher, JM Holden, DB Haytowitz, SE Gebhardt, and RL Prior. "Lipophilic and hydrophilic antioxidant capacities of common foods in the United States." *Journal of Agricultural and Food Chemistry* 52(12) (2004): 4026–37.

Lambert, JD, S Sang, and CS Yang. "Possible controversy over dietary polyphenols: Benefits vs risks." *Chemical Research In Toxicology* 20(4) (2007): 583–585.

Yoto, A, M Motoki, S Murao, and H Yokogoshi. "Effects of L-theanine or caffeine intake on changes in blood pressure under physical and psychological stresses." *Journal of Physiological Anthropology* 31(1) (2012): 28.

National Cancer Institute. "Tea And Cancer Prevention: Strengths And Limits Of The Evidence." National Institute of Health. 2010 (Internet). www.cancer.gov/cancertopics/factsheet/prevention/tea.

Ferruzzi, MG. "The influence of beverage composition on delivery of phenolic compounds from coffee and tea." *Physiology & Behavior* 100(1) (2010): 33–41.

Schwalfenberg, G, SJ Genuis, and I Rodushkin. "The benefits and risks of consuming brewed tea: beware of toxic element contamination." *Journal of Toxicology* 2013 (2013): Article ID 370460.

CHAPTER 3

Kim A, A Chiu, MK Barone, D Avino, F Wang, CI Coleman, et al. "Green tea catechins decrease total and low-density lipoprotein cholesterol: a systematic review and metaanalysis." *Journal of the American Dietetic Association* 111(11) (2011): 1720–9.

Liu, K, R Zhou, B Wang, K Chen, LY Shi, JD Zhu, et al. "Effect of green tea on glucose control and insulin sensitivity: a meta-analysis of 17 randomized controlled trials." *American Journal of Clinical Nutrition* 98(2) (2013): 340–8.

Shkayeva, MV, et al. "Green tea product epigallocatechin gallate (EGCG) content and label information: a descriptive analysis." *Journal of Nutritional Therapeutics* 4(3) (2015): 81–84.

Steptoe, A, et al. "The effects of tea on psychophysiological stress responsivity and post-stress recovery: a randomised double-blind trial." *Psychopharmacology* 190(1) (2007): 81–89.

Ilya C, W Arts, et al. "Catechin contents of foods commonly consumed in the Netherlands." *Journal of Agricultural and Food Chemistry* 48(5) (2000): 1752–1757.

Venditti, Elisabetta et al. "Hot vs. cold water steeping of different teas: Do they affect antioxidant activity?" *Food Chemistry* 119 (2010): 1597–1604.

Inoue, M, et al. "Regular consumption of green tea and the risk of breast cancer recurrence: follow-up study from the Hospital-based Epidemiologic Research Program at Aichi Cancer Center (HERPACC), Japan." *Cancer Letters* 167(2) (2001): 175–82.

Kurahashi, N, et al. "Green tea consumption and prostate cancer risk in Japanese men: a prospective study." *American Journal of Epidemiology* 167(1) (2007): 71-7.

CHAPTER 4

Beliveau R, and D Gingras. "Green tea: prevention and treatment of cancer by nutraceuticals." *Lancet* 364(9439) (2004): 1021-2.

Weiss, DJ, and CR Anderton. "Determination of catechins in matcha green tea by micellar electrokinetic chromatography." *Journal of Chromatography* 1011(1-2) (2003): 173–80.

Dulloo, AG, C Duret, D Rohrer, L Girardier, N Mensi, M Fathi, P Chantre, and J Vandermander. "Efficacy of a green tea extract rich in catechin polyphenols and caffeine in increasing 24-h energy expenditure and fat oxidation in humans." *American Journal of Clinical Nutrition* 70(6) (1999): 1040-5.

Nagao, T, et al. "Ingestion of a tea rich in catechins leads to a reduction in body fat and malondialdehyde-modified LDL in men." *American Journal of Clinical Nutrition* 81(1) (2005): 122-9.

Khokhar, S, and S Magnusdottir. "Total phenol, catechin, and caffeine contents of teas commonly consumed in the United Kingdom." *Journal of Agricultural and Food Chemistry* 50(3) (2002): 565-70.

Weiss, DJ, and DR Anderton. "Determination of catechins in matcha green tea by micellar electrokinetic chromatography." *Journal of Chromatography A.* 1011(1-2) (2003): 173–80.

Zheng, XX, YL Xu, et al. "Green tea intake lowers fasting serum total and LDL cholesterol in adults: a meta-analysis of 14 randomized controlled trials." *American Journal of Clinical Nutrition* 94(2) (2011): 601-10.

Komes, D, et al. "Green tea preparation and its influence on the content of bioactive compounds." *Food Research International* 43 (1) (2010): 167–176.

CHAPTER 5

Duffy, SJ, et al. "Short- and long-term black tea consumption reverses endothelial dysfunction in patients with coronary artery disease." Cirulation 104 (2001) 151–156.

Thomas, JA, L Gerber, LL Banez, DM Moreira, RS Rittmaster, GL Andriole, and SJ Freedland. "Prostate Cancer Risk in Men with Baseline History of Coronary Artery Disease: Results from the REDUCE study." *Cancer Epidemiology, Biomarkers, & Prevention* 21(4) (2012): 576–81.

Rasmussen-Torvik, LJ, CM Shay, JG Abramson, CA Friedrich, JA Nettleton, AE Prizment, and AR Folsom. "Ideal cardiovascular health is inversely associated with incident cancer: the atherosclerosis risk in communities study." *Circulation* 127 (2013): 1270–1275.

Tokunaga S, IR White, C Frost, K Tanaka, S Kono, S Tokudome, T Akamatsu, T Moriyama, and H Zakouji. "Green tea consumption and serum lipids and lipoproteins in a population of healthy workers in Japan." *Annals of Epidemiology* 12(3) (2002): 157–65.

Hopkins AL, et al. "Hibiscus sabdariffa L. in the treatment of hypertension and hyperlipidemia: a comprehensive review of animal and human studies." *Fitoterapia* 85 (2013): 84–94.

Hertog, MGL, et al. "Flavonoid intake and long-term risk of coronary heart disease and cancer in the seven countries study." *Archives of Internal Medicine* 155(4) (1995): 381–386.

Alexopoulos, N, et al. "The acute effect of green tea consumption on endothelial function in healthy individuals." *European Journal of Cardiovascular Prevention & Rehabilitation* 15(3) (2008): 300.

Grassi, D, TPJ Mulder, R Draijer, G Desideri, H Molhuizen, and C Ferri. "Black tea consumption dose-dependently improves flow-mediated dilation in healthy males." *Journal of Hypertension* 27(4) (2009): 774–781.

CHAPTER 6

Maki, KC, et al. "Green tea catechin consumption enhances exercise-induced abdominal fat loss in overweight and obese adults." *Journal of Nutrition* 139(2) (2009): 264–70.

Lin, JK, and SY Lin-Shiau. "Mechanisms of hypolipidemic and anti-obesity effects of tea and tea polyphenols." *Molecular Nutrition & Food Research* 50(2) (2006): 211–217.

Venables, MC, CJ Hulston, et al. "Green tea extract ingestion, fat oxidation, and glucose tolerance in health humans." *American Journal of Clinical Nutrition* 87 (2008): 778–84.

Kao, YH, RA Hiipakka, and S Liao. "Modulation of obesity by a green tea catechin." *American Journal of Clinical Nutrition* 72(5) (2000): 1232–4.

Hara, Y. *Green tea: health benefits and applications.* New York: Marcel Dekker, pp. 139–148, 2001.

Furuyashiki, T, H Nagayasu, Y Aoki, H Bessho, T Hashimoto, K Kanazawa, and H Ashida. "Tea catechin suppresses adipocyte differentiation accompanied by down-regulation of PPARY2 and C/EBPa in 3T3-L1 cells." *Bioscience, Biotechnology, and Biochemistry* 68(11) (2004): 2353–2359.

Koo, SI, and SK Noh. "Green tea as inhibitor of the intestinal absorption of lipids: potential mechanism for its lipid-lowering effect." *Journal of Nutritional Biochemistry* 18(3) (2007): 179–183.

Hase, T, Y Komine, S Meguro, Y Takeda, H Takahasci, Y Matsui, S Inaoka, Y Katsuragi, I Tokimitsu, H Shimasaki, and H Itakura. "Anti-obesity effects of tea catechins in humans." *Journal of Oleo Science* 50 (2001): 599–605.

Venables, MC, CJ Hulston, , HR Cox, and AE Jeukendrup. "Green tea extract ingestion, fat oxidation and glucose tolerance in healthy humans." *American Journal of Clinical Nutrition* 87 (2008): 778–84.

Westerterp-Plantenga, MS, MP Lejeune, and EM Kovacs. "Body weight loss and weight maintenance in relation to habitual caffeine intake and green tea supplementation." *Obesity Research & Clinical Practice* 13(7) (2005): 1195–204.

Maggio CA, and FX Pi-Sunyer. "The prevention and treatment of obesity. Application to type 2 diabetes." *Diabetes Care* 20(11) (1997): 1744–66.

Nakai, M, Y Fukui, S Asami, Y Toyoda-Ono, T Iwashita, H Shibata, T Mitsunaga, F Hashimoto, and Y Kiso. "Inhibitory effects of oolong tea polyphenols on pancreatic lipase in vitro." *Journal of Agricultural and Food Chemistry* 53(11) (2005): 4593–8.

Grossmann, ME, A Ray, KJ Nkhata, DA Malakhov, OP Rogozina, S Dogan, and MP Cleary. "Obesity and breast cancer: status of leptin and adiponectin in pathological processes." *Cancer and Metastasis Review* 29(4) (2010): 641–53.

Kelesidis, I, T Kelesidis, and CS Mantzoros. "Adiponectin and cancer: a systematic review." *British Journal of Cancer* 94 (2006): 1221–1225.

van Kruijsdijk, RCM, E van der Wall, and FVisseren. "Obesity and cancer: the role of dysfunctional adipose tissue." *Cancer Epidemiology, Biomarkers & Prevention* 18 (2009): 2569.

Kelly, T, W Yang, C-S Chen, K Reynolds, and J He. "Global burden of obesity in 2005 and projections to 2030." *International Journal of Obesity* 32 (2008): 1431–1437.

Arent, SM, et al. "The effects of theaflavin-enriched black tea extract on muscle soreness, oxidative stress, inflammation, and endocrine responses to acute anaerobic interval training: a randomized, double-blind, crossover study." *Journal of the International Society of Sports Nutritionists* 7 (2010): 11.

CHAPTER 7

Barrett, B, et al. "Meditation or exercise for preventing acute respiratory infection: a randomized controlled trial." *Annals of Family Medicine* 10(4) (2012): 337–346.

Steptoe A, EL Gibson, R Vuononvirta, ED Williams, M Hamer, JA Rycroft, JD Erusalimsky, and J Wardle. "The effects of tea on psychophysiological stress responsivity and post-stress recovery: a randomised double-blind trial." *Psychopharmacology* 190(1) (2007): 81–9.

Keenan, E, M Finnie, P Jones, P Rogers, and C Priestle. "How much theanine in a cup of tea? Effects of tea type and method of preparation." *Food Chemistry* 125 (2011): 588–594.

Comstock, GW, et al. "Cardiovascular risk factors in American and Japanese executives. Telecom Health Research Group." *Journal of the Royal Society of Medicine* 78 (1985): 536–45.

Juneja, LR, et al. "L-theanine—a unique amino acid of green tea and its relaxation effect in humans." *Trends in Food Science & Technology* 10 (1999): 199–204.

Kobayashi, K, et al. "Effects of L-theanine on the release of brain waves in human volunteers." *Nippon Noegik Kaishi* 72 (1998): 153–57.

Sadakata, S, et al. "Mortality among female practitioners of Chanoyu (Japanese "tea-ceremony")." *Tohoku Journal of Experimental Medicine* 166 (1992): 475–77.

Sesso, HD, et al. "Coffee and tea intake and the risk of myocardial infarction." *American Journal of Epidemiology* 149 (1999): 162–7.

Simons, LA, et al. "Health status and lifestyle in elderly Hawaii Japanese and Australian men. Exploring known differences in longevity." *Medical Journal of Australia* 157 (1992): 188–90.

Nieoullon, A ."Dopamine and the regulation of cognition and attention." *Progress in Neurobiology* 67(1) (2002): 53–83.

Moreno-Smith, M, SK Lutgendorf, and AK Sood. "Impact of stress on cancer metastasis." *Future Oncology* 6(12) 2010: 1863–1881.

Hai, T, CC Wolford, and YS Chang. "ATF3, a hub of the cellular adaptive-response network, in the pathogenesis of diseases: is modulation of inflammation a unifying component?" *Gene Expression* 15(1) 2010: 1–11.

Welsh, J, M Meagher, and EM Sternberg, Editors. *Neural and neuroendocrine mechanisms in host defense and autoimmunity.* Kluwer Press, 2006.

Sapolsky, RM. Why Zebras Don't Get Ulcers: A Guide to Stress, Stress-Related Diseases, and Coping. WH Freeman and Co.; NY, USA: 1998.

Chrousos G. "Stress and disorders of the stress system." *Nature Reviews Endocrinology* 5 (2009): 374–381.

McEwen, B. "Stressed or stressed out: What is the difference?" *Journal of Psychiatry & Neuroscience* 30(5) (2005): 315–318.

CHAPTER 8

Cohen, S, and TA Willis. "Stress, social support, and the buffering hypothesis." *Psychological Bulletin* 98 (1985): 310–357.

Reynolds P, and GA Kaplan. "Social connections and risk for cancer: prospective evidence from the Alameda County study." *Behavioral Medicine* 16(3) (1990): 101–10.

Moreno-Smith, M, SK Lutgendorf, and AK Sood. "Impact of stress on cancer metastasis." *Future Oncology* 6(12) 2010: 1863–1881.

Funch, DP, and J Marshall. "The role of stress, social support and age in survival from breast cancer." *Journal of Psychosomatic Research* 27 (1983): 77–83.

Marshall, JR, and DP Funch. "Social environment and breast cancer. A cohort analysis of patient survival." *Cancer* 52(8) (1983): 1546–1550.

Maunsell, E, J Brisson, and L Deschenes. "Social support and survival among women with breast cancer." *Cancer* 76(4) (1995): 631–637.

Yang, YC, C Boen, K Gerken, T Li, K Schorpp, and K Mullan Harris. "Social relationships and physiological determinants of longevity across the human life span." *Proceedings of the National Academy of Sciences*, 2016: 201511085

Emmons, R. *How the New Science of Gratitude Can Make You Happier* (Houghton Mifflin, 2007)

Algoe, SB. "Find, remind, and bind: the functions of gratitude in everyday relationships." *Social and Personality Psychology Compass* 6(6) (2012).

ACKNOWLEDGMENTS

Like everything in life, this book was a gift. Many thanks to Elizabeth Seise and Will Kiester of Page Street Publishing for this project, which has become a chapter of its own in my story. It's been joyful, inspiring and challenging, and would never have come to fruition without the loving help and support from so many.

THANK YOU TO

* My amazing husband, Donald, for your unbridled love and the freedom you give me to chase my dreams with passion.

* My most loving daughters, Anna and Laura, for inspiring me to be a better person, by example, and reminding me daily what we are made of.

* My marvelous colleagues—Jessica, Shaunna, Jane, Mary, Hope, Jackie, Jordan, Daniela, Octavio, Conci, Andy and Elsy—for your persistent excellence and support, sprinkled with humor and joyfulness, on our path to fostering health and wellness by infusing the goodness of tea.

* Hope and Mary—For your talents for flavors and ingenuity in recipe development and testing.

* Hope, Ted, Elise and Laura—Your insights and talents have shaped this book, and your fabric is woven throughout its pages—giving it structure, illustration and sparkle.

ABOUT THE AUTHOR

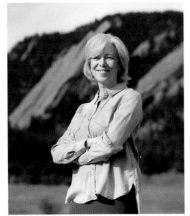

Maria Uspenski is the founder of The Tea Spot, a leading producer of craft teas, based in Boulder, Colorado. The philanthropic company's mission is to advance healthier living through the everyday enjoyment of whole leaf tea. The Tea Spot donates 10 percent of all sales in-kind to cancer and community wellness.

Maria's love of tea was fostered at an early age by her Russian family. Later, as an undergraduate student in Paris she was introduced to many more varieties than the traditional black teas of her childhood. During stints as a ballet dancer and athlete, Maria began to discover the health benefits of tea. It is her core belief that loose leaf tea can be made simple enough for the every day and that even the most inexperienced tea drinker should be enjoying and infusing tea in its purest, whole leaf form.

A Massachusetts Institute of Technology mechanical engineer by education, Maria is the The Tea Spot's innovative force, listed on three U.S. patents for Steepware inventions, which promote the ease of tea preparation. Her message is simple and powerful—tea in its freshest form is not only sustainable and delicious, it is a powerful elixir with unmatched health benefits.

Maria has been featured in the Huffington Post and on television interviews for her success as a social entrepreneur, cancer fighter and certified tea and fitness nutrition expert. She has been a regular contributor to blogs for *The Denver Post*, T-Ching and The Tea Spot, and is called on to lecture about the health benefits of tea at universities and conferences nationwide. Maria lives in the mountains of Colorado, with her husband, Don.

INDEX